Updates in Surgery

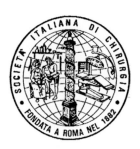

Luigi Angrisani
Editor

Bariatric and Metabolic Surgery

Indications, Complications and Revisional Procedures

In collaboration with
Maurizio De Luca, Giampaolo Formisano,
and Antonella Santonicola

Forewords by
Francesco Corcione
Enrico Di Salvo

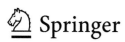 Springer

Editor
Luigi Angrisani
General and Endoscopic Surgery Unit
S. Giovanni Bosco Hospital
Naples, Italy

The publication and the distribution of this volume have been supported by the Italian Society of Surgery

ISSN 2280-9848
Updates in Surgery
ISBN 978-88-470-3943-8

ISSN 2281-0854 (electronic)

ISBN 978-88-470-3944-5 (eBook)

DOI 10.1007/ 978-88-470-3944-5

Springer Milan Dordrecht Heidelberg London New York

Library of Congress Control Number: 2016943835

© Springer-Verlag Italia S.r.l. 2017

Cover design: eStudio Calamar S.L.
External publishing product development: Scienzaperta, Novate Milanese (Milan), Italy
Typesetting: Graphostudio, Milan, Italy

This Springer imprint is published by Springer Nature
Springer-Verlag Italia S.r.l. – Via Decembrio 28 – I-20137 Milan
Springer is a part of Springer Science+Business Media (www.springer.com)

Foreword

Twenty years ago, some surgeons considered bariatric surgery to be equivalent to experimental surgery. However, over the last 20 years this surgery has had a wide diffusion thanks to professional, economic and ethical interests. The reason for this rapid spread can be found in the increasing demand for surgical treatments that may save patients from morbid and disabling obesity. Patients seek a solution to their problem after having tested a variety of treatments, and they turn to surgery as their last resort.

Since the early, exclusively laparotomic, experiences of the pioneer Prof. Scopinaro, many minimally invasive procedures have been introduced – such as Scopinaro's biliopancreatic diversion, gastric banding, sleeve gastrectomy and other procedures each with specific indications – in order to be able to offer obese patients a tailored surgery as is the case with other pathologies.

Owing to its complexity, this type of surgery has required the institution of a multidisciplinary team for the treatment of all aspects of morbid obesity. A new scientific Society was set up which rapidly became the point of reference for the entire scientific community.

For these reasons, after the historical biennial conference of Prof. Basso, the Italian Society of Surgery had to take into consideration this type of surgery with its implications in term of complications, redo surgery and results.

In this context, Prof. Angrisani, a pioneer of bariatric surgery and president of the major International Society of Bariatric Surgery, has had a central role because of his experience and dedication. Bariatric surgery has taken advantage of technological improvements, and the laparoscopic approach has become routine in this field. I am grateful to Prof. Angrisani and the other speakers for the task they have accomplished with great commitment and dedication.

I would also like to thank Springer, as always and more than ever, for their organizational effectiveness and editorial expertise in assisting my distinguished colleagues in this report.

Rome, September 2016
Francesco Corcione
President, Italian Society of Surgery

Foreword

Bariatric, or weight loss, surgery is a recent surgical specialty that aims to reduce weight-related disorders and improve quality of life. Weight loss procedures, like transplant surgery, require specific knowledge and skill, while the patient's anthropometric and psychological peculiarities demand an adequate multidisciplinary approach.

Originating in the world's richest countries, surgery for obesity and weight-related diseases gradually spread across the developing world as a consequence of the obesity and diabetes epidemic.

Modern lifestyles are characterized by an incorrect balance between calorie intake and energy expenditure, leading to increased body weight and excess adipose tissue. Excess body fat is a threat to patients' health as well as undermining their self-esteem and social life. As a result, the treatment of these patients requires not only a skilled surgeon but also an expert medical and psychological team.

Since bariatric surgeons, more than other doctors, operate on patients at particularly high risk, they should adequately inform their patients and strictly follow the international guidelines on the indications for surgery.

For these reasons, increasing numbers of young surgeons should start studying and practising bariatric surgery, to improve the medical and surgical treatment of obesity. The importance of this surgical specialty has too often been underestimated, while the clinical, social and economic benefits of weight loss procedures cannot be denied or ignored in modern medicine.

This book was conceived as a guide to help the various specialists and professionals (surgeons, internists, dieticians, diabetologists, psychologists, etc.) understand the importance of this discipline, the only one able to treat the current epidemic of obesity and weight-related diseases. A further aim is to promote a wider knowledge of bariatric surgery techniques, outcomes and complications among general surgeons.

Naples, September 2016

Enrico Di Salvo
Professor of General Surgery
Federico II University of Naples, Italy

Preface

Obesity is considered a multifactorial disease that results from a combination of genetic predisposition, environmental influences (e.g., sedentary lifestyle), and behavioral components. Obesity has become a pandemic affecting billions of people worldwide. Being overweight and obese are well-known causes of morbidity and mortality, with significant health, social and economic implications, due to the cost of the many comorbidities that are often associated.

Bariatric surgery is currently considered the most effective treatment option for morbid obesity. When compared with nonsurgical interventions, bariatric surgery results in greater improvements not only in weight loss outcomes but also in obesity-related comorbidities. The aim of bariatric surgery has therefore been upgraded from a merely weight-loss surgery to a metabolic surgery. Different surgical options are currently available and they are continuously evolving under the influence of the literature results, specific local conditions, and the experience of the surgical staff in each country.

Through 20 chapters this book offers a summary of all the aspects of bariatric and metabolic surgery, illustrating the evolution of bariatric surgery in Italy and worldwide and describing the indications, surgical technique, and complications of all the most commonly performed bariatric procedures. Unfortunately, a certain percentage of the operations performed is associated with inadequate weight loss or anatomic complications due to multiple concurrent factors. Therefore, bariatric surgeons are now routinely facing an increasing number of patients who need a second or third obesity procedure: the so-called "revisional surgery". In fact, three chapters are dedicated to this topic and deal with the clinical and surgical management of this emerging class of patients. Last chapters focus on some "hot topics" in bariatric surgery – such as diabetes surgery and the problem of gastroesophageal reflux disease and hiatal hernia – and provide an overview of the endoluminal procedures and some other bariatric procedures.

A wide range of healthcare professionals (bariatric surgeons, general surgeons, psychologists, and gastroenterologists) have been involved in the writing of these chapters because I firmly believe that a multidisciplinary team is essential for the management of obesity.

I would like to express my gratitude to all the colleagues who contributed to the preparation of this book, which will hopefully serve as a useful manual for a wide range of healthcare professionals.

Naples, September 2016   Luigi Angrisani

Contents

1 History of Obesity Surgery in Italy 1
Vincenzo Pilone, Ariola Hasani, Giuliano Izzo, Antonio Vitiello,
and Pietro Forestieri

2 Current Indications to Bariatric Surgery in Adult, Adolescent,
and Elderly Obese Patients 9
Luca Busetto, Paolo Sbraccia, and Ferruccio Santini

3 Bariatric Surgery Worldwide 19
Luigi Angrisani, Giampaolo Formisano, Antonella Santonicola,
Ariola Hasani, and Antonio Vitiello

4 Evolution of Bariatric Surgery in Italy: Results of the
National Survey 25
Nicola Di Lorenzo, Giuseppe Navarra, Vincenzo Bruni,
Ida Camperchioli, and Luigi Angrisani

5 Gastric Banding 31
Maurizio De Luca, Gianni Segato, David Ashton, Cesare Lunardi,
and Franco Favretti

6 Sleeve Gastrectomy 41
Emanuele Soricelli, Giovanni Casella, Alfredo Genco, and Nicola Basso

7 Roux-en-Y Gastric Bypass 57
Cristiano Giardiello, Pietro Maida, and Michele Lorenzo

8 Mini-Gastric Bypass/One Anastomosis Gastric Bypass 69
Maurizio De Luca, Emilio Manno, Mario Musella, and Luigi Piazza

9 Standard Biliopancreatic Diversion 79
Nicola Scopinaro, Giovanni Camerini, and Francesco S. Papadia

10 Duodenal Switch   93
Gianfranco Silecchia, Mario Rizzello, and Francesca Abbatini

11 Single Anastomosis Duodenoileal Bypass with Sleeve Gastrectomy . . 107
Luigi Angrisani, Ariola Hasani, Antonio Vitiello, Giampaolo Formisano,
Antonella Santonicola, and Michele Lorenzo

12 Ileal Interposition   117
Diego Foschi, Andrea Rizzi, and Igor Tubazio

13 The Problem of Weight Regain   127
Roberto Moroni, Marco Antonio Zappa, Giovanni Fantola,
Maria Grazia Carbonelli, and Fausta Micanti

14 Band Revision and Conversion to Other Procedures   137
Vincenzo Borrelli and Giuliano Sarro

15 Sleeve Revision and Conversion to Other Procedures   143
Mirto Foletto, Alice Albanese, Maria Laura Cossu, and Paolo Bernante

16 RYGB Revision and Conversion to Other Procedures   151
Daniele Tassinari, Rudj Mancini, Rosario Bellini, Rossana Berta,
Carlo Moretto, Abdul Aziz Sawilah, and Marco Anselmino

**17 The Problem of Gastroesophageal Reflux Disease
and Hiatal Hernia**   165
Paola Iovino, Antonella Santonicola, and Luigi Angrisani

18 Diabetes Surgery: Current Indications and Techniques   173
Paolo Gentileschi, Stefano D'Ugo, and Francesco Rubino

19 Endoluminal Procedures   183
Giovanni Domenico De Palma, Alfredo Genco, Massimiliano Cipriano,
Gaetano Luglio, and Roberta Ienca

20 Other Bariatric Procedures   195
Marcello Lucchese, Stefano Cariani, Enrico Amenta, Ludovico Docimo,
Salvatore Tolone, Francesco Furbetta, Giovanni Lesti,
and Marco Antonio Zappa

All web addresses have been checked and were correct at time of printing.

Contributors

Francesca Abbatini Department of Medico-Surgical Sciences and Biotechnologies, Division of General Surgery and Bariatric Center, Sapienza University of Rome, Latina, Italy

Alice Albanese Center for the Study and the Integrated Management of Obesity, Department of Medicine, University Hospital of Padua, Padua, Italy

Enrico Amenta University of Bologna, Bologna, Italy

Luigi Angrisani General and Endoscopic Surgery Unit, S. Giovanni Bosco Hospital, Naples, Italy

Marco Anselmino Bariatric and Metabolic Surgery Unit, Azienda Ospedaliera-Universitaria Pisana, Pisa, Italy

David Ashton Imperial College School of Medicine, Birmingham, United Kingdom

Nicola Basso Department of Surgical Sciences, Sapienza University of Rome, Rome, Italy

Rosario Bellini Bariatric and Metabolic Surgery Unit, Azienda Ospedaliera-Universitaria Pisana, Pisa, Italy

Paolo Bernante General Surgery Unit, Civic Hospital, Pieve di Cadore, Italy

Rossana Berta Bariatric and Metabolic Surgery Unit, Azienda Ospedaliera-Universitaria Pisana, Pisa, Italy

Vincenzo Borrelli General and Bariatric Surgery Unit, Istituto di Cura Città di Pavia, Gruppo Ospedaliero San Donato, Pavia, Italy

Vincenzo Bruni Belcolle Public Hospital, Viterbo, Italy

Luca Busetto Center for the Study and the Integrated Management of Obesity, Department of Medicine, University Hospital of Padua, Padua, Italy

Giovanni Camerini Department of Surgery, University of Genoa Medical School, Genoa, Italy

Ida Camperchioli Department of Experimental Medicine and Surgery, University of Rome Tor Vergata, Rome, Italy

Maria Grazia Carbonelli Dietology and Nutrition Unit, Medical Surgical Department, AO San Camillo Forlanini, Rome, Italy

Stefano Cariani Obesity Surgery Center, Digestive Tract Diseases and Internal Medicine Department, Bologna University Hospital, Bologna, Italy

Giovanni Casella Department of Surgical Sciences, Sapienza University of Rome, Rome, Italy

Massimiliano Cipriano Department of Surgical Sciences, Sapienza University of Rome, Rome, Italy

Maria Laura Cossu General Surgery Unit, Department of Clinical and Experimental Medicine, University of Sassari, Sassari, Italy

Maurizio De Luca Department of Surgery, Montebelluna Treviso Hospital, Montebelluna, Italy

Giovanni Domenico De Palma Department of Clinical Medicine and Surgery, University of Naples Federico II, Naples, Italy

Nicola Di Lorenzo Department of Experimental Medicine and Surgery, University of Rome Tor Vergata, Rome, Italy

Ludovico Docimo General and Bariatric Surgery Unit, Department of Medical, Surgical, Neurological, Metabolic and Ageing Sciences, Second University of Naples, Naples, Italy

Stefano D'Ugo Department of Surgery, University of Rome Tor Vergata, Rome, Italy

Giovanni Fantola Bariatric Surgery Unit, Department of Surgery, AO Brotzu, Cagliari, Italy

Franco Favretti Department of Surgery, Casa di Cura Eretenia, Vicenza, Italy

Mirto Foletto Center for the Study and the Integrated Management of Obesity, Department of Medicine, University Hospital of Padua, Padua, Italy

Pietro Forestieri Department of Clinical Medicine and Surgery, University of Naples Federico II, Naples, Italy

Giampaolo Formisano Division of General and Minimally Invasive Surgery, Misericordia Hospital, Grosseto, Italy

Diego Foschi Department of Biomedical Sciences Luigi Sacco, University of Milan, Milan, Italy

Franceso Furbetta General, Endoscopic and Bariatric Surgery, Clinica Leonardo, Sovigliana-Vinci, Italy

Alfredo Genco Department of Surgical Sciences, Multidisciplinary Center for the Treatment of Obesity, Policlinico Umberto I University Hospital, Sapienza University of Rome, Rome, Italy

Paolo Gentileschi Bariatric Surgery Unit, University of Rome Tor Vergata, Rome, Italy

Cristiano Giardiello General, Emergency and Metabolic Surgery Unit, Department of Surgery and Obesity Center, Pineta Grande Hospital, Castelvolturno, Italy

Ariola Hasani Department of Clinical Medicine and Surgery, University of Naples Federico II, Naples, Italy

Roberta Ienca Department of Experimental Medicine, Sapienza University of Rome, Rome, Italy

Paola Iovino Gastrointestinal Unit, Department of Medicine and Surgery, University of Salerno, Salerno, Italy

Giuliano Izzo Department of Clinical Medicine and Surgery, University of Naples Federico II, Naples, Italy

Giovanni Lesti Fondazione Salus, Bariatric Center, Clinica Di Lorenzo, Avezzano, Italy

Michele Lorenzo Forensic Medicine Unit, Distretto 56, ASL Napoli 3 Sud, Torre Annunziata, Italy

Marcello Lucchese General, Metabolic and Emergency Unit, Department of Surgery, Santa Maria Nuova Hospital, Florence, Italy

Gaetano Luglio Department of Clinical Medicine and Surgery, University of Naples Federico II, Naples, Italy

Cesare Lunardi Department of Surgery, Montebelluna Treviso Hospital, Montebelluna, Italy

Pietro Maida General Surgery Unit, Center of Oncologic and Advanced Laparoscopic Surgery, Evangelical Hospital Villa Betania, Naples, Italy

Rudj Mancini Bariatric and Metabolic Surgery Unit, Azienda Ospedaliera-Universitaria Pisana, Pisa, Italy

Emilio Manno Department of Surgical Sciences, Cardarelli Hospital, Naples, Italy

Fausta Micanti Department of Neuroscience, Reproductive Science and Odontostomatology, School of Medicine Federico II, Naples, Italy

Carlo Moretto Bariatric and Metabolic Surgery Unit, Azienda Ospedaliera-Universitaria Pisana, Pisa, Italy

Roberto Moroni Bariatric Surgery Unit, Department of Surgery, AO Brotzu, Cagliari, Italy

Mario Musella General Surgery, Department of Advanced Biomedical Sciences, University of Naples Federico II, Naples, Italy

Giuseppe Navarra Department of Human Pathology of Adult and Evolutive Age, University Hospital of Messina, Messina, Italy

Francesco S. Papadia Department of Surgery, University of Genoa Medical School, Genoa, Italy

Luigi Piazza General Surgery Unit, ARNAS Garibaldi, Catania, Italy

Vincenzo Pilone Department of Medicine and Surgery, University of Salerno, Salerno, Italy

Mario Rizzello Department of Medico-Surgical Sciences and Biotechnologies, Division of General Surgery and Bariatric Center, Sapienza University of Rome, Latina, Italy

Andrea Rizzi Department of General Surgery, Luigi Sacco Hospital, Milan, Italy

Francesco Rubino Metabolic and Bariatric Surgery, Division of Diabetes and Nutritional Sciences, King's College London, London, United Kingdom

Ferruccio Santini Obesity Center, Endocrinology Unit, University Hospital of Pisa, Pisa, Italy

Antonella Santonicola Gastrointestinal Unit, Department of Medicine and Surgery, University of Salerno, Salerno, Italy

Giuliano Sarro Department of General Surgery, Cesare Cantù Hospital of Abbiategrasso, Abbiategrasso, Italy

Abdul Aziz Sawilah Bariatric and Metabolic Surgery Unit, Azienda Ospedaliera-Universitaria Pisana, Pisa, Italy

Paolo Sbraccia Department of Systems Medicine, University of Rome Tor Vergata, and Obesity Center, University Hospital Policlinico Tor Vergata, Rome, Italy

Nicola Scopinaro Department of Surgery, University of Genoa Medical School, Genoa, Italy

Gianni Segato Department of Surgery, S. Bortolo Regional Hospital, Vicenza, Italy

Gianfranco Silecchia Department of Medico-Surgical Sciences and Biotechnologies, Division of General Surgery and Bariatric Center, Sapienza University of Rome, Latina, Italy

Emanuele Soricelli Department of Surgical Sciences, Sapienza University of Rome, Rome, Italy

Daniele Tassinari Bariatric and Metabolic Surgery Unit, Azienda Ospedaliera-Universitaria Pisana, Pisa, Italy

Salvatore Tolone General and Bariatric Surgery Unit, Department of Medical, Surgical, Neurological, Metabolic and Ageing Sciences, Second University of Naples, Naples, Italy

Igor Tubazio Department of General Surgery, Luigi Sacco Hospital, Milan, Italy

Antonio Vitiello Department of Clinical Medicine and Surgery, University of Naples Federico II, Naples, Italy

Marco Antonio Zappa Department of General and Emergency Surgery, Sacra Famiglia Fatebenefratelli Hospital, Erba, Italy

History of Obesity Surgery in Italy

1

Vincenzo Pilone, Ariola Hasani, Giuliano Izzo, Antonio Vitiello, and Pietro Forestieri

1.1 Epidemiology of Obesity in Italy

Overweight and obesity rates are constantly increasing in industrialized countries. In 2013, according to statistical data, more than one out of ten Italian adults (11.3%) is obese, while 34.5% of the population is overweight [1]. However, the latest data show that the proportion of overweight adults has only mildly increased since the early 2000s and the rate has been stabilizing in recent years. In this context, southern regions have a higher prevalence of obesity; for example, the obese population in Puglia represents 13.6% compared with 9% in Lombardia, and the overweight population is 39.2% in Campania compared with 30% in Trentino-Alto Adige [1].

1.2 Early Years of Bariatric Surgery

Bariatric surgery in Italy began in early 1970, a time when obesity was still considered worldwide as being the consequence of an inappropriate lifestyle and not a serious multifactorial disease. In 1972 in Milan, Montorsi [2–5] performed the first jejunoileal bypass (JIB) following a long period of research on obesity and its related pathologies. He was a pioneer not only as a bariatric surgeon but as a physician, since he understood that a multidisciplinary approach was the only effective way to achieve success in the treatment of obese patients. In the same period intense bariatric research took place in different Italian institutions by different groups: Montorsi and Doldi in Milan, Battezzati and Scopinaro in

A. Vitiello (✉)
Department of Clinical Medicine and Surgery, University of Naples Federico II
Naples, Italy
e-mail: antoniovitiello_@hotmail.it

L. Angrisani (Ed), Bariatric and Metabolic Surgery,
Updates in Surgery
DOI: 10.1007/ 978-88-470-3944-5_1, © Springer-Verlag Italia 2017

Genoa, Mazzeo and Forestieri in Naples, Morino and Toppino in Turin, Grassi and Santoro in Rome, Vecchioni and Baggio in Verona, and Vassallo in Pavia. The initial experience with JIB showed good outcomes with acceptable compliance but also unsatisfactory weight loss and catastrophic results such as liver failure, bypass enteritis, and excessive weight loss with severe malnutrition requiring reintervention. Media and medical societies firmly opposed this surgery, inducing some bariatric surgeons to abandon the practice and others to find new solutions. In Genoa in 1973, Scopinaro [6–9] began his first series of JIB and at the same time ideated and experimented with a new procedure on animals – biliopancreatic diversion (BPD) – performed for the first time on humans on 12 May 1976. The procedure consisted of a distal gastrectomy with a long-limb Roux-en-Y reconstruction and an enteroenteric anastomosis performed in the terminal ileum. BPD was conceived in an attempt to avoid complications associated with JIB, which were primarily due to the presence of the long blind loop, non-selective malabsorption, and intestinal adaptation syndrome. What Scopinaro observed on animals was then confirmed in patients: BPD seemed to solve the primary problems associated with JIB. Scopinaro represents a milestone in the history of bariatric surgery worldwide, not only as a surgeon but also for his important studies on intestinal physiology, which allowed better comprehension of intestinal absorption. Different techniques were developed as variations or simplifications of the Scopinaro procedure, thus confirming that BPD still represents one of the most effective bariatric procedures, even after 40 years. Mazzeo and Forestieri [10] in Naples performed the first series of JIB in 1974, at a time when many authors reported weight regain likely due to the alimentary reflux in the excluded loop. In an attempt to solve this side effect, Forestieri [11] ideated the end-to-side jejunoileostomy with an antireflux valve system, the successful outcomes of which were presented at the Biennial World Congress of the International College of Surgeons in Athens, Greece, in 1976. This modification resulted in extensive application worldwide, and Forestieri [12, 13] was the first Italian surgeon cited in the history of the evolution of bariatric surgery, published by Buchwald [14]. In Turin in 1975, Morino began his bariatric experience with the JIB, and after inconsistent results, in 1978, he adopted the Roux-en-Y gastric bypass and, in 1983, Mason's vertical gastroplasty. In Rome, after evaluating the outcomes of his own extensive experience with JIB, Santoro was one of the first authors to describe postoperative adaptation syndrome and bypass intolerance syndrome [15–18].

In 1979, the School of Montorsi performed the first biliointestinal bypass in Italy in an attempt to reduce the effects of bacterial overgrowth in the blind loop and malabsorption of bile salts. In 1990, Doldi definitively adopted the biliointestinal bypass as the standard procedure in obese patients who were candidates for malabsorptive procedures.

In Bologna, in 1991, Amenta and Cariani [19–21] began their bariatric experience with Mason's vertical gastroplasty, and later in 1996, they adopted the laparoscopic Roux-en-Y gastric bypass (LRYGB) procedure. After constant research and clinical activity, in 2002, they introduced a modification to preserve the possibility of endoscopically and radiologically evaluating the excluded gastroenteric tract: the Roux-en-Y gastric bypass on vertical banded gastroplasty (Amenta-Cariani), which is still the standard procedure in their center for treating obesity. In 1997, in Pavia, Vassallo [22] introduced an evolution of BPD: BPD coupled with transitory gastroplasty, which preserves the duodenal bulb. The gastroplasty is transitory due to the use of a biodegradable polydioxanone (PDS) band.

The enthusiastic bariatric activity and the need to gather and share experiences led Italian bariatric surgeons create the Italian Society of Bariatric Surgery (SICOB) in Genoa in 1991 and, with Carlo Vassallo, to the institution of the first School of Bariatric Surgery, entrusted to the Associazione Chirurghi Ospedalieri Italiani (ACOI). SICOB is one of five founding societies of the International Federation for the Surgery of Obesity and Metabolic Disorders (IFSO) and the first bariatric society in the world to add the concept of metabolic surgery to its name, changing it to Society of Bariatric and Metabolic Surgery in 2007.

1.3 The Beginning of Laparoscopy

Italians surgeons have always been pioneers in the surgical treatment of obesity and weight-related diseases. In the early 1990s, they began proposing and adopting several endoscopic and laparoscopic procedures. In 1993, for the first time worldwide, Catona [23] placed a silicone gastric band laparoscopically; the same year, Favretti [24] performed the first laparoscopic adjustable gastric banding (LAGB), which allowed placement of the posterior aspect of the band in the thickness of the mesogastrium, thus creating an extremely small (virtual) anterior gastric pouch. This perigastric intervention was the initial gold standard technique for LAGB. Later, a different approach – the pars flaccida technique – gained popularity, since it is more effective in preventing slippage and other complications after band placement [25, 26].

In the mid-1990s, many other bariatric centers began their experience with LAGB, which rapidly became the most frequently performed gastric bypass procedure in Italy. Satisfactory results of LAGB on specific patients, such as the superobese, those with low body mass index (BMI), and the elderly individuals, were accomplished and the results published before they were reported by other countries. The Italian Group for Lap-Band still leads international guidelines and perspectives due to the extensive knowledge accumulated over the past 15 years.

In 1995, Catona [27] performed the first videolaparoscopic vertical banded gastroplasty (LVBG), and in 2002, Morino [28] published a series of 250 cases showing that LVBG was an effective and safe procedure in morbidly obese patients, providing good weight loss with a low morbidity rate and minimum discomfort. However, in superobese patients, LVBG was questionable, and more complex procedures were taken into account. As with open surgery, the laparoscopic approach allowed the creation of a calibrated transgastric window using a circular stapler and the fashioning of a linear gastric pouch along the lesser curve using a linear stapler. The operation was completed by positioning a polypropylene band at the distal part of the gastric pouch. In 2001, Forestieri et al. [29, 30] demonstrated that success following use of the BioEnterics Intragastric Balloon (BIB) in patients undergoing LAGB was predictive of weight loss after banding (BIB test). Success of adjustable banding in Italy and other industrialized countries was definitely due to the feasibility of using the laparoscopic approach. On the other hand, the diffusion of laparoscopy in bariatric surgery was certainly induced by the satisfactory outcomes of LAGB. However, it did not take long for Italian surgeons to begin performing more advanced procedures using a minimally invasive approach.

1.4   The Modern Era

At the beginning of the third millennium, the extensive knowledge gained regarding surgical treatment of obesity and the laparoscopic experience with restrictive procedures also induced many surgeons to perform laparoscopically procedures that were more complex than LAGB. Several centers began performing LRYGB at approximately the same time (it is indeed difficult to establish who was the first). In 2007, Angrisani et al. [31] were the first to report their 5-year outcomes with LRYGB, which resulted in better weight loss and a reduced number of failures compared with LAGB, despite the significantly longer operative time and possible life-threatening complications.

Italian bariatric surgeons have also proposed and performed laparoscopic modifications of the traditional gastric bypass technique. In June 2001, Lesti [32] designed and performed the first laparoscopic gastric bypass with fundectomy and exploration of the remnant stomach. The idea was to remove the gastric fundus and create a passage between the pouch and the remnant stomach, which can therefore be investigated endoscopically. At the same time, Furbetta [33] designed a new procedure: the functional gastric bypass (FGB). In this technique, a gastric band is positioned around the upper part of the stomach, with the addition of a hand-sewn side-to-side gastroenterostomy between the gastric pouch and the small bowel in the form of an omega loop. Inflation or deflation of the band allows activation or deactivation of the bypass. In 2006, Parini [34] et al. published their outcomes with robotic Roux-en-Y gastric bypass using the Da Vinci robot-assisted approach. The authors found that the performance of gastrojejunostomy anastomosis using the robot is easier and the results more certain than with the same laparoscopic procedure, because it is performed with the help of a tridimensional view and restored hand–eye coordination.

The first experience with laparoscopic malabsorptive surgery was published by Scopinaro [35, 36] in 2002, who described the technique and reported early results of laparoscopic biliopancreatic diversion (LBPD). In 2003, the same authors described in detail their experience with 42 patients using a retrocolic submesocolic approach to create a gastroenteroanastomosis.

The biliopancreatic diversion with duodenal switch (BPD-DS) [37, 38] was initially performed with a two-stage approach, creating a "sleeve" resection of the stomach as the first step. This laparoscopic sleeve gastrectomy (LSG) was intended to reduce operative risk (American Society of Anesthesiologists score) in superobese patients undergoing bariatric surgery. In 2006, Basso et al. [39, 40] were the first to publish their experience showing that LSG alone represented a safe and effective procedure to achieve marked weight loss as well as significantly reduce major obesity-related comorbidities. The authors found that using this approach caused a reduction of ghrelin, thus providing a metabolic effect as well. As for LAGB, in the early period of laparoscopy, the effectiveness and feasibility of LSG induced many centers to prefer this procedure over LRYGB and LBPD.

The ability of Italian bariatric surgeons to foresee new and promising procedures is demonstrated by the recent success of the laparoscopic mini-gastric bypass (LMGB). This new intervention, following a similar trend in the United States, has raised doubt concerning the risk of determining biliary gastritis and cancer of the gastric pouch in the long term. In June 2012, despite skepticism, LMGB was approved in Italy by SICOB, and a multicenter retrospective study claiming its effectiveness has already been carried out [41]. Although bariatric surgery in Italy is continuously moving toward new frontiers, we cannot find a better way to conclude this brief history than citing the godfather of this discipline, Nicola Scopinaro: "Only the long experience, culture, dedication of professionals who really do this surgery with the only aim of giving these unfortunate patients hope for the future can guarantee the correct use of bariatric operations."

References

1. ISTAT - Istituto Nazionale di Statistica (2014) Condizioni di salute e ricorso ai servizi sanitari. Anno 2013. Parte seconda - Fattori di rischio e prevenzione. 2.2 Sovrappeso e obesità (Tavole 2.2.1–2.2.5) http://www.istat.it/it/files/2014/12/tavoledicembre.zip?title=La+salute+e+il+ricorso+ai+servizi+sanitari+-+29%2Fdic%2F2014+-+Tavole.zip
2. Montorsi W, Doldi SB (1981) Surgical treatment of massive obesity: our experience with jejuno-ileal bypass. World J Surg 5:801–806
3. Doldi SB, Montorsi W (1984) Jejuno-ileal latero-lateral bypass. Defects of mechanical sutures. Presse Med 13:1571–1572 [Article in French]
4. Montorsi W, Doldi SB, Klinger R, Montorsi F (1986) Surgical therapy for morbid obesity. Int Surg 71:84–86
5. Doldi SB, Lattuada E, Zappa MA et al (1998) Biliointestinal bypass: another surgical option. Obes Surg 8:566–569

6. Scopinaro N, Gianetta E, Berretti B, Caponnetto A (1976) A case of severe obesity treated jejunoileal bypass: 1-year clinical course. Minerva Chir 31:341–359

7. Scopinaro N, Gianetta E, Civalleri D et al (1979) The biliopancreatic bypass for functional surgical treatment of obesity. Minerva Med 70:3537–3547

8. Scopinaro N, Gianetta E, Civalleri D et al (1979) Bilio-pancreatic bypass for obesity: I. An experimental study in dogs. Br J Surg 66:613–617

9. Scopinaro N, Gianetta E, Civalleri D et al (1979) Bilio-pancreatic bypass for obesity: II. Initial experience in man. Br J Surg 66:618–620

10. Mazzeo F, Forestieri P, De Luca L (1977) Risultati del bypass digiuno-ileale termino-laterale. Atti del III Congresso Nazionale dell'Unione Italiana contro l'Obesità. Società Editrice Universo, Roma

11. Forestieri P, De Luca L, Mazzeo F, Scrocca A (1976) End-to-side jejuno-ileal bypass in the treatment of gross obesity: a modified Payne technique. Abstracts from Proceedings of the XX Biennial World Congress of the International College of Surgeons

12. Forestieri P, De Luca L, Bucci L, Mazzeo F (1977) Surgical treatment of high degree obesity. Our own criteria to choose the appropriate type of jejuno-ileal bypass. A modified Payne technique. Chirurgia Gastroenterologica 11:401–405

13. Forestieri P, Formisano C, Bucci L et al (1984) Surgical therapy of severe obesity: results and complications. Our experience with termino-lateral jejuno-ileal bypass (personal method). Minerva Chir 39:1307–1314 [Article in Italian]

14. Buchwald H (2014) The evolution of metabolic/bariatric surgery. Obes Surg 24:1126–1135

15. Grassi G, Cantarelli I, Dell'Osso A (1975) Intestinal bypass in the treatment of severe obesity. Personal experience. Chirurgie 101:920–927 [Article in French]

16. Santoro E, Allegri C, Ciaraldi F (1977) A new technique of jejuno-ileal anastomosis for the treatment of morbid obesity. Surg Italy 7:126–132

17. Santoro E, Allegri C, Garofalo A (1980) Special gastric bypass in associated diabetes and obesity. Chirurgia Generale 1:167–169

18. Santoro E et al (1984) Gastroplastiche e by pass gastro-enterici nella cura chirurgica della grande obesità. G Chir 5:124–127

19. Cariani S, Amenta E (2007) Three-year results of Roux-en-Y gastric bypass-on-vertical banded gastroplasty: an effective and safe procedure which enables endoscopy and X-ray study of the stomach and biliary tract. Obes Surg 17:1312–1318

20. Cariani S, Palandri P, Della Valle E et al (2008) Italian multicenter experience of Roux-en-Y gastric bypass on vertical banded gastroplasty: four-year results of effective and safe innovative procedure enabling traditional endoscopic and radiographic study of bypassed stomach and biliary tract. Surg Obes Relat Dis 4:16–25

21. Cariani S, Agostinelli L, Leuratti L et al (2009) Roux en-Y gastric bypass on vertical banded gastroplasty (variante Amenta-Cariani): risultati a 5 anni di follow-up. Osp Ital Chir 15:421–431

22. Vassallo C, Negri L, Della Valle A et al (1997) Biliopancreatic diversion with transitory gastroplasty preserving duodenal bulb: 3 years' experience. Obes Surg 7:30–33

23. Catona, A, Gossenberg M, La Manna A, Mussini G (1993) Laparoscopic gastric banding: preliminary series. Obes Surg 3:207–209

24. Favretti F, Cadiere GB, Segato G et al (1995) Laparoscopic adjustable gastric banding (LAP-BAND): technique and results. Obes Surg 5:364–371

25. Angrisani L, Lorenzo M, Esposito G et al (1997) Laparoscopic adjustable silicone gastric banding: preliminary results of the University of Naples experience. Obes Surg 7:19–21

26. Morino M, Toppino M, Garrone C (1997) Disappointing long-term results of laparoscopic adjustable silicone gastric banding. Br J Surg 84:868–869

27. Catona A, Gossenberg M, Mussini G et al (1995) Videolaparoscopic vertical banded gastroplasty. Obes Surg 5:323–326

28. Morino M, Toppino M, Bonnet G et al (2002) Laparoscopic vertical banded gastroplasty for morbid obesity: assessment of efficacy. Surg Endosc 16:1566–1172

29. Genco A, Bruni T, Doldi SB et al (2005) BioEnterics Intragastric Balloon: the Italian experience with 2,515 patients. Obes Surg 15:1161–1164

30. Loffredo A, Cappuccio M, De Luca M et al (2001) Three years experience with the new intragastric balloon, and a preoperative test for success with restrictive surgery. Obes Surg 11:330–333

31. Angrisani L, Lorenzo M, Borrelli V (2007) Laparoscopic adjustable gastric banding versus Roux-en-Y gastric bypass: 5-year results of a prospective randomized trial. Surg Obes Relat Dis 3:127–132

32. Lesti G (2015) Tecnica del by-pass gastrico sec. Lesti. Oral communication at XXIII SICOB National Congress, Baveno (Italy)

33. Furbetta F, Gambinotti G (2002) Functional gastric bypass with an adjustable gastric band. Obes Surg 12:876–880

34. Parini U, Fabozzi M, Brachet Contul R et al (2006) Laparoscopic gastric bypass performed with the Da Vinci Intuitive Robotic System: preliminary experience. Surg Endosc 20:1851–1857

35. Scopinaro N, Marinari GM, Camerini G (2002) Laparoscopic standard biliopancreatic diversion: technique and preliminary results. Obes Surg 12:241–244

36. Camerini G, Marinari GM, Scopinaro N (2003) A new approach to the fashioning of the gastro-entero anastomosis in laparoscopic standard biliopancreatic diversion. Surg Laparosc Endosc Percutan Tech 13:165–167

37. Cossu ML, Noya G, Tonolo GC et al (2004) Duodenal switch without gastric resection: results and observations after 6 years. Obes Surg 14:1354–1359

38. Mittempergher F, Bruni T, Bruni O et al (2002) Biliopancreatic diversion with preservation of the duodenal bulb and transitory gastroplasty in the treatment of morbid obesity: our experience. Ann Ital Chir 73:137–142

39. Silecchia G, Boru C, Pecchia A et al (2006) Effectiveness of laparoscopic sleeve gastrectomy (first stage of biliopancreatic diversion with duodenal switch) on co-morbidities in super-obese high-risk patients. Obes Surg 16:1138–1344

40. Basso N, Casella G, Rizzello M et al (2011) Laparoscopic sleeve gastrectomy as first stage or definitive intent in 300 consecutive cases. Surg Endosc 25:444–449

41. Musella M, Susa A, Greco F et al (2014) The laparoscopic mini-gastric bypass: the Italian experience: outcomes from 974 consecutive cases in a multicenter review. Surg Endosc 28:156–163

Current Indications to Bariatric Surgery in Adult, Adolescent, and Elderly Obese Patients

Luca Busetto, Paolo Sbraccia, and Ferruccio Santini

2.1 Introduction

Indications for obesity surgery were for the first time formalized in 1991 [1]. Since then and until recently, indications remained substantially unchanged worldwide. In recent years, however, the accrual of new data on the efficacy and safety of obesity surgery in patients not originally included in the first indications, coupled with the growing burden of obesity epidemics and the still unmet need for nonsurgical weight loss strategies, opened the way to several attempts to revise original criteria. In this chapter, previous and novel guidelines for bariatric surgery are revised in the context of new clinical and epidemiologic data.

2.2 Bariatric Surgery in Adults

The prevalence of obesity in adults is increasing worldwide. According to the World Health Organization (WHO) Global Database on Body Mass Index (BMI), 39% of adults (age ≥18 years) were overweight and 13% were obese in 2014 [2]. Prevalence of obesity varies greatly across the WHO regions, being much more prevalent in the Americas, in Europe, and in the eastern Mediterranean region. The global prevalence of obesity has nearly tripled since 1980 [2], configuring an unprecedented "epidemic" for a noncommunicable disease. An even greater increase has occurred for the most severe forms of obesity. Whereas the general prevalence of obesity (BMI >30 kg/m²) doubled in the last 15 years of the

L. Busetto (✉)
Center for the Study and the Integrated Management of Obesity, Department of Medicine, University Hospital of Padua
Padua, Italy
e-mail: luca.busetto@unipd.it

L. Angrisani (Ed), Bariatric and Metabolic Surgery,
Updates in Surgery
DOI: 10.1007/ 978-88-470-3944-5_2, © Springer-Verlag Italia 2017

twentieth century in the USA, the prevalence of morbid obesity (BMI >40 kg/m²) had a four-fold increase and the prevalence of superobesity (BMI >50 kg/m²) had a six-fold increase [3].

As stated, indications for obesity surgery were for the first time formalized in 1991, at the very beginning of the obesity epidemics, when obesity surgery had a very limited diffusion and was still in an early stage of development. The 1991 guidelines were formalized by an expert consensus conference endorsed by the US National Institutes of Health (NIH) and contained a statement on criteria for patient selection [1]. The guidelines, purely based on expert opinion, indicated bariatric surgery in morbidly obese patients fulfilling the following criteria:

- BMI >40 kg/m² (or BMI >35 kg/m² with comorbid conditions)
- age groups from 18 to 60 years
- obesity lasting >5 years
- patients who failed to lose weight or to maintain long-term weight loss despite appropriate nonsurgical medical care
- patient willingness to participate in a postoperative multidisciplinary treatment program.

Comorbid conditions for which patients with BMI 35–40 kg/m² could be indicated to bariatric surgery were not clearly specified in the 1991 guidelines. However, they were generally considered as conditions significantly contributing to morbidity and mortality in obese patients and in which surgically induced weight loss is expected to improve the disorder (such as metabolic disease, cardiorespiratory disease, disabling joint disease, and others).

Contraindications for bariatric surgery reported in the 1991 document [1], and constantly confirmed thereafter, can be summarized as follows:

- absence of a period of identifiable medical management
- patients unable to participate in prolonged medical follow-up
- psychotic disorders, severe depression, and personality and eating disorders
- alcohol abuse and/or drug dependencies
- diseases threatening life in the short term
- patients unable to care for themselves and have no adequate family or social support.

Despite the fact that the 1991 indications were not supported by any evidence-based result at the time of their release, they subsequently proved to be clinically reasonable according to results obtained in long-term controlled studies. The most important long-term study in bariatric surgery is the Swedish Obese Subjects (SOS) study, a controlled trial that compared the outcome of 2000 patients who underwent bariatric surgery by various techniques with that of a matched control group that received conventional treatment [4]. In the surgery group, the average 10-year weight loss from baseline stabilized at 16.1%, whereas in controls, the average weight during the observation period increased by 1.6%. This substantial difference in weight loss was associated with significant differences in relevant clinical outcomes. Cumulative overall mortality in the surgery group was 34% lower than that observed in controls [5], the incidence of fatal and nonfatal first-time cardiovascular events was 33% lower [6], the number of first-time cancers was 42% lower in women [7], and the incidence of new cases of diabetes mellitus (DM) was 83% lower [4]. In patients already having type 2 DM at enrollment, the DM remission rate 2 years after surgery was 16.4% in controls and 72.3% in the surgery group [8]. Despite the fact that type 2 DM tends to relapse over time in >50% of surgical patients having short-term remission, the cumulative incidence of microvascular and macrovascular complications was, respectively, 56% and 32% lower in the surgical group than in the control group [8].

The general contents of the NIH 1991 guidelines have been repeatedly and, until recently, confirmed in several international documents (ACC/AHA/TOS 2013; NICE 2014; IFSO-EC/EASO 2014) [9–11], with only minimal changes and specifications. In particular, according to the National Institute for Health and Clinical Excellence (NICE) 2014 guidelines, recognized failure of a previous nonsurgical treatment program may not be strictly required in patients with extremely high BMI (>50 kg/m^2) [10]. As for BMI criterion, it is important to note that a documented previous high BMI should be considered, meaning that weight loss as a result of intensified preoperative treatment is not a contraindication for the planned bariatric surgery, even if patients reach a BMI below that required for surgery. Furthermore, bariatric surgery is indicated in patients who exhibited substantial weight loss following a conservative treatment program but started to regain weight [11].

The first attempt at opening the way to bariatric surgery in some patients having a BMI below the usual boundaries for indication was in patients with type 2 DM. This significant and still debated step was stimulated by accumulating evidences about the efficacy and safety of modern bariatric surgery in diabetic patients with mild obesity (BMI 30–35 kg/m^2). In particular, groups of patients with these characteristics were included in some of the randomized, controlled, clinical trials comparing bariatric surgery and conventional treatment in obese patients with type 2 DM. First, Dixon et al. randomized obese patients (BMI 30–40 kg/m^2) with recently diagnosed type 2 DM to gastric banding or conventional therapy with a focus on weight loss. At 2-year follow-up, remission of DM was achieved in 73% patients in the surgical group and 13% in the conventional-therapy group [12]. More recently, Schauer et al. randomized obese patients (BMI 27–43 kg/m^2) with uncontrolled type 2 DM to receive either intensive medical therapy alone or intensive medical therapy plus gastric bypass or sleeve gastrectomy in the STAMPEDE (Surgical Treatment and Medications Potentially Eradicate Diabetes Efficiently) trial. The primary endpoint was a glycated hemoglobin (HbA1c) level of ≤6.0%. At 3 years, the target was achieved in 5% of patients in the medical-therapy group compared with 38% of those in the gastric-bypass group and 24% of those in the sleeve-gastrectomy group. Both weight loss and glycemic control were greater in the surgical groups than in the medical-therapy group [13]. Finally, Ikramuddin et al. randomized obese diabetic patients (BMI 30–40 kg/m^2) to receive intensive medical management or gastric bypass plus an intensive lifestyle-medical management protocol. The primary endpoint was a composite goal of HbA1c ≤7.0%, low-density lipoprotein cholesterol ≤100 mg/dL, and systolic blood pressure ≤130 mmHg. At 12 months, 49% of patients in the gastric bypass group and 19% in the lifestyle-medical management group achieved the composite goal [14]. The results observed in these small randomized trials have been confirmed in several prospective and retrospective studies specifically dedicated to the application of bariatric surgery in diabetic patients with BMI <35 kg/m^2 [15, 16]. A direct comparison among these studies is difficult because of substantial differences in inclusion criteria, primary procedures, and definition of therapeutic goals. However, the overall message is a confirmation of the superiority of bariatric surgery over medical therapy in producing an improvement of metabolic control and/or achieving remission of type 2 DM in patients with mild obesity, without substantial differences with respect to results observed in patients with more severe obesity forms.

The first official position in favor of the use of bariatric surgery in patients with type 2 DM and mild obesity was held by the International Diabetes Federation (IDF) in 2011 [17]. The IDF suggested that bariatric surgery should be considered in diabetic patients with BMI 30–35 kg/m^2 when DM cannot be adequately controlled by optimal medical regimen, especially in the presence of other major cardiovascular disease risk factors [17]. More recently, the 2013 clinical practice guidelines of the American Association of Clinical Endocrinologists, the Obesity Society, and the American Society for Metabolic and Bariatric Surgery, suggested that a bariatric procedure may be offered to patients with BMI 30–34.9 kg/m^2 and with DM or metabolic syndrome [18]. Taking into account the common observation of a higher probability of DM remission after surgery in patients with a shorter DM history, the NICE 2014 obesity guidelines suggested bariatric surgery in patients with mild obesity and recent-onset type 2 DM [10]. Finally, application of bariatric surgery to diabetic patients with BMI 30–35 kg/m^2 is permitted on an individual basis in the recent Interdisciplinary European Guidelines on Metabolic and Bariatric Surgery [11] and the European Guidelines for Obesity Management in Adults [19]. However, it should be noted that this opening to the application of bariatric surgery in diabetic patients with a BMI level below the traditional limits for surgery is not uniformly accepted. In particular, the 2014 American Diabetes Association (ADA) Standards of Medical Care in Diabetes [20] confirmed that although small trials have shown glycemic benefit of bariatric surgery in patients with type 2 DM and BMI 30–35 kg/m^2, there is currently insufficient evidence to generally recommend surgery in patients with BMI <35 kg/m^2). Particular emphasis has been posed regarding the lack of long-term data demonstrating net benefit in this particular group of patients [18–20].

Apart from type 2 DM, a case in favor of the use of obesity surgery has been raised also for patients with mild obesity suffering from other severe obesity-related health problems. The superiority of bariatric surgery over a lifestyle-medical management program in inducing weight loss and improving comorbid conditions has been demonstrated in nondiabetic patients with moderate obesity

(BMI 30–35 kg/m^2) by a small randomized, controlled trial with a 2-year follow-up [21]. On the basis of these results, the Clinical Issue Committee of the American Society for Metabolic and Bariatric Surgery recommended that for patients with BMI 30–35 kg/m^2 who do not achieve substantial and durable weight and comorbidity improvement with nonsurgical methods, bariatric surgery should be an available option [22].

The question of the eventual inclusion of patients with mild obesity in surgical treatment protocols should be viewed in the context of the present criticism to the pivotal role of BMI levels in guiding therapeutic decisions. The simple use of BMI can be misleading in clinical practice, taking into account that BMI calculation is only a proxy for fat-mass measurement and that the relationships between BMI levels and the occurrence of obesity-related comorbidities is imprecise. An effort in favor of a better characterization or phenotyping of obese patients, well beyond simple BMI levels, is urgently advocated [23]. In this context, a recent position statement from the International Federation for the Surgery of Obesity and Metabolic Disorders regarding bariatric surgery in class I obesity highlighted the inadequacy of the simple BMI value as an indicator of the clinical state and comorbidity burden in the obese patient [24]. The document emphasized the common clinical observation that patients with relatively low BMI values may have a comorbidity burden similar to or greater than patients with more severe obesity and concluded that denial of bariatric surgery to obese patients with BMI 30–35 kg/m^2 suffering from severe comorbidities and not achieving weight control with nonsurgical therapy does not appear to be clinically justified [24]. However, it should be emphasized that long-term results describing the risk/benefit ratio of bariatric surgery in patients with moderate obesity (with or without DM) are not available; therefore, potential risks related to excessive weight loss should be considered with caution in this category of patients.

2.3   Bariatric Surgery in Adolescents

Obesity trends in children and adolescents mimicked trends of the obesity epidemic observed in adults, and the alarming prevalence of obesity has been observed at young ages in several countries worldwide. In this age group, the aggressive campaign against obesity and unhealthy dietary pattern seems to have achieved initial positive results. Among US children and adolescents aged 2–19 years, obesity prevalence stabilized between 2003 and 2004 and 2011 and 2012 overall (−0.2 percentage points), with a significant decrease among 2- to 5-year-old US children (−5.5 percentage points) [25]. Data from other countries have also shown a decline or stabilization of obesity levels in children. Despite this encouraging progress, the global situation remains alarming. In 2011–2012, the prevalence of obesity in the United States was 16.9% in individuals 2 to 19 years [25]. In Italy, 22.2% of children in primary school were overweight, and 10.6% were obese in 2012, with even worst figures in the southern regions of the country [26]. Obesity epidemics in children and adolescents substantially challenged pediatric medicine, which is now facing complications once typical only of adulthood: insulin resistance, type 2 DM, dyslipidemia, nonalcoholic fatty liver disease, metabolic syndrome, hypertension [27]. These complications are associated in children and adolescents with cardiovascular events, cancer, and premature death, as in adults [27]. Obese children are also at higher risk of precocious puberty, polycystic ovary syndrome, sleep apnea, orthopedic complications, and psychological and social disturbances [28]. Finally, obese children have a higher probability of becoming obese adults, thus fueling the current epidemic of obesity and related diseases [28].

The NIH 1991 guidelines did not suggest the use of bariatric surgery in the severely obese population <18 year old [1], and young patients have had limited access to the procedure for many years. However, under pressure of the dramatic increase in obesity in young people, bariatric surgery for adolescents has been progressively increasing, with results undergoing careful and complete review [29], including a randomized controlled trial. O'Brien et al. compared bariatric surgery (gastric banding) with a lifestyle intervention program in a small group of adolescents 14–18 years of age and BMI >35 kg/m². The authors confirmed the superiority of bariatric surgery at 2-year follow-up in terms of weight loss and improvement in comorbidities and quality of life (QoL) [30]. The efficacy and safety of bariatric surgery in adolescents was recently tested in the Teen-Longitudinal Assessment of Bariatric Surgery (Teen-LABS) study, a prospective clinical and laboratory study of teenagers undergoing gastric bypass and sleeve gastrectomy at five centers in the United States. At 3 years after the procedure, mean weight decreased by 27%, with significant improvements in cardiometabolic health and weight-related QoL [31].

The paucity of reliable data regarding the efficacy and safety of bariatric surgery in children and adolescents resulted in more stringent indication criteria than those applied to adults. According to the Interdisciplinary European Guidelines on Metabolic and Bariatric Surgery [11], and in agreement with the recommendations of a consensus document of American pediatricians [32], in adolescents with severe obesity, bariatric surgery can be considered if the patient meets the following conditions:

- BMI >40 kg/m² (or 99.5th percentile for respective age) and at least one comorbidity
- followed at least 6 months of organized weight-reducing attempts in a specialized center
- shows skeletal and developmental maturity
- is capable of committing to comprehensive medical and psychological evaluation before and after surgery
- is willing to participate in a postoperative multidisciplinary treatment program.

However, on the base of new knowledge, it now seems reasonable to move the indications for bariatric surgery in adolescents closer to those used in adults. Recently proposed selection criteria are as follows [29]:

- BMI >35 kg/m^2 and serious comorbidities (type 2 DM, moderate or severe obstructive sleep apnea [apnea-hypopnea index (AHI) >15 events/h), pseudotumor cerebri, and severe steatohepatitis]
- BMI >40 kg/m^2 and another comorbidity [mild obstructive sleep apnea (AHI ≥5 events/h), hypertension, insulin resistance, glucose intolerance, dyslipidemia, impaired QoL or activities of daily living]
- Tanner stage IV or V (unless severe comorbidities indicate bariatric surgery earlier)
- skeletal maturity of at least 95% of estimated growth
- ability to understand what dietary and physical activity changes will be required for optimal postoperative outcomes
- evidence of mature decision making, with appropriate understanding of potential risks and benefits of surgery
- evidence of appropriate social support without evidence of abuse or neglect
- appropriate treatment of possible coexisting psychiatric conditions (depression, anxiety, or binge-eating disorder)
- evidence that family and patient have the ability and motivation to comply with recommended treatments pre- and postoperatively, including consistent use of micronutrient supplements; evidence may include a history of reliable attendance at office visits for weight management and compliance with other medical needs.

The procedures for which there is enough evidence to recommend bariatric surgery for adolescents are gastric banding [30], gastric bypass [31], and sleeve gastrectomy [31]. It is usually recommended that the procedure be performed in highly specialized centers with extensive multidisciplinary experience and pediatric surgical skills [11].

2.4   Bariatric Surgery in the Elderly

The prevalence of obesity in the elderly is increasing in Western countries. Data from the National Health and Nutrition Examination Survey (NHANES 2011–2012) showed that in the US population, the prevalence of obesity in people >60 years was 32% in men and 38% in women [25]. The association between obesity and morbidity (hypertension, dyslipidemia, glucose intolerance, type 2 DM, cardiovascular diseases) in younger adults is maintained in the older population [33]. Moreover, obesity is now recognized as an important disability factor in the elderly [34].

The NIH 1991 guidelines did not suggest the use of bariatric surgery in severely obese individuals >60 years [1]. However, those guidelines were written in a time when obesity surgery was in a very early stage of development, was mostly conducted as open surgery, and had a relatively high surgical risk. Moreover, the problem of obesity in the elderly was not appreciated at that time. The advent of the laparoscopic approach reduced the risk and greatly improved postsurgery recovery. On the other hand, the increase in life span coupled with advances in modern medicine considerably increased the number of patients with a very long lifespan. Preventing obesity-related disability in this large population has become one of the major challenges in obesity treatment in several countries [33]. Over the same period, some initial experiences with bariatric surgery in elderly patients began to report satisfactory results [35–40]. Generally, these studies were conducted in patients between 60 and 70 years old who were in good clinical and physical condition. The studies reported a slightly greater incidence of postoperative complications and lower weight loss compared with younger patients yet displaying advantages in terms of improvement or remission of comorbid conditions and amelioration of functional autonomy and QoL.

Ultimately, bariatric surgery can be considered for patients >60 years and who have indications similar to those applied in the younger adult patient after a careful individual estimate of risks and benefits and with the primary aim being the potential improvement in QoL and the patient's functional status [11, 33].

2.5   Conclusions

In conclusion, available data confirm the safety and efficacy of bariatric surgery in adult patients with severe obesity. Technical progress in bariatric surgery and growing scientific evidence now suggest that surgery could be a valid therapeutic options in patients for which it was not originally indicated, such those with mild obesity but severe obesity-related health burden, obese adolescents, and obese elderly patients with good functional status and long life expectancy.

References

1. National Institutes of Health (1991) Gastrointestinal surgery for severe obesity. National Institutes of Health Consensus Development Conference Draft Statement. Obes Surg 1:257–265
2. World Health Organization (2015) Obesity and overweight. Fact sheet No 311. http://www.who.int/topics/obesity/en
3. Sturm R (2003) Increases in clinically severe obesity in the United States, 1986-2000. Arch Intern Med 163:2146–2148
4. Sjöström L (2013) Review of the key results from the Swedish Obese Subjects (SOS) trial – a prospective controlled intervention study of bariatric surgery. J Intern Med 273 219–234
5. Sjöström L, Narbro K, Sjöström CD et al (2007) Swedish Obese Subjects Study: effects of bariatric surgery on mortality in Swedish obese subjects. N Engl J Med 357:741–752

6. Sjöström L, Peltonen M, Jacobson P et al (2012) Bariatric surgery and long-term cardiovascular events. JAMA 307:56–65
7. Sjöström L, Gummesson A, Sjöström CD et al (2009) Effects of bariatric surgery on cancer incidence in obese patients in Sweden (Swedish Obese Subjects Study): a prospective, controlled intervention trial. Lancet Oncol 10:653–662
8. Sjöström L, Peltonen M, Jacobson P et al (2014) Association of bariatric surgery with long-term remission of type 2 diabetes and with microvascular and macrovascular complications. JAMA 311:2297–304
9. American College of Cardiology/American Heart Association Task Force on Practice Guidelines, Obesity Expert Panel, 2013 (2014) Executive summary: Guidelines (2013) for the management of overweight and obesity in adults: a report of the American College of Cardiology/American Heart Association Task Force on Practice Guidelines and the Obesity Society published by the Obesity Society and American College of Cardiology/American Heart Association Task Force on Practice Guidelines. Based on a systematic review from the The Obesity Expert Panel, 2013. Obesity (Silver Spring) 22(Suppl 2):S5–S39
10. National Institute for Health and Clinical Excellence (2014) Obesity: identification, assessment and management of overweight and obesity in children, young people and adults. NICE clinical guideline CG189. https://www.nice.org.uk/guidance/cg189
11. Fried M, Yumuk V, Oppert JM et al on behalf of International Federation for the Surgery of Obesity and Metabolic Disorders - European Chapter and European Association for the Study of Obesity (2014) Interdisciplinary European guidelines on metabolic and bariatric surgery. Obes Surg 24:42–55
12. Dixon JB, O'Brien PE, Playfair J et al (2008) Adjustable gastric banding and conventional therapy for type 2 diabetes: a randomized controlled trial. JAMA 299:316–23
13. Schauer PR, Bhatt DL, Kirwan JP et al (2014) Bariatric surgery versus intensive medical therapy for diabetes - 3-Year outcomes. N Engl J Med 370:2002–2013
14. Ikramuddin S, Korner J, Lee WJ et al (2013) Roux-en-Y gastric bypass vs intensive medical management for the control of type 2 diabetes, hypertension, and hyperlipidemia: the Diabetes Surgery Study randomized clinical trial. JAMA 309:2240–2249
15. Li Q, Chen L, Yang Z et al (2012) Metabolic effects of bariatric surgery in type 2 diabetic patients with body mass index <35 kg/m². Diabetes Obes Metab 14:262–270
16. Reis CE, Alvarez-Leite JI, Bressan J, Alfenas RC (2012) Role of bariatric–metabolic surgery in the treatment of obese type 2 diabetes with body mass index <35 kg/m²: a literature review. Diabetes Technol Ther14:365–372
17. Dixon JB, Zimmet P, Alberti KG et al (2011) Bariatric surgery: an IDF statement for obese type 2 diabetes. Diabet Med 28:628–642
18. Mechanick JI, Youdim A, Jones DB et al (2013) Clinical practice guidelines for the perioperative nutritional, metabolic, and nonsurgical support of the bariatric surgery patient–2013 update: cosponsored by American Association of Clinical Endocrinologists, the Obesity Society, and American Society for Metabolic and Bariatric Surgery. Surg Obes Relat Dis 9:159–191
19. Yumuk V, Tsigos C, Fried M et al for the Obesity Management Task Force of the European Association for the Study of Obesity (2015) European guidelines for obesity management in adults. Obes Facts 8:402–424
20. American Diabetes Association (2014) Standards of medical care in diabetes – 2014. Diabetes Care 37(Suppl 1):S14–S80
21. O'Brien PE, Dixon JB, Laurie C et al (2006) Treatment of mild to moderate obesity with laparoscopic adjustable gastric banding or an intensive medical program. A randomized trial. Ann Intern Med 144:625–633
22. ASMBS Clinical Issues Committee (2013) Bariatric surgery in class I obesity (BMI 30–35 kg/m²). Surg Obes Relat Dis 9:e1–e10
23. Blundell JE, Dulloo AG, Salvador J, Frühbeck G (2014) EASO SAB Working Group on BMI. Beyond BMI–phenotyping the obesities. Obes Facts 7:322–328

24. Busetto L, Dixon J, De Luca M et al (2014) Bariatric surgery in class I obesity: a Position Statement from the International Federation for the Surgery of Obesity and Metabolic Disorders (IFSO). Obes Surg 24:487–519
25. Ogden CL, Carroll MD, Kit BK, Flegal KM (2014) Prevalence of childhood and adult obesity in the United States, 2011-2012. JAMA 311:806–814
26. Istituto Superiore di Sanità (2016) Il Sistema di sorveglianza OKkio alla SALUTE: risultati 2014 (a cura di Nardone P, Spinelli A, BuoncristianoM et al). ISS, Rome. http://www.iss.it/binary/publ/cont/ONLINE_Okkio.pdf
27. Weiss R, Dziura J, Burgert TS et al (2004) Obesity and the metabolic syndrome in children and adolescents. N Engl J Med 350:2362–2374
28. Han JC, Lawlor DA, Kimm SYS (2010) Childhood obesity. Lancet 375:1737–1748
29. Pratt JSA, Lenders CM, Dionne EA et al (2009) Best practice updates for pediatric/adolescent weight loss surgery. Obesity (Silver Spring) 17:901–910
30. O'Brien PE, Sawyer SM, Laurie C et al (2010) Laparoscopic adjustable gastric banding in severely obese adolescents. A randomized trial. JAMA 303:519–526
31. Inge TH, Courcoulas AP, Jenkins TM et al for the Teen-LABS Consortium (2016) Weight loss and health status 3 years after bariatric surgery in adolescents. N Engl J Med 374:113–123
32. Inge TH, Krebs NF, Garcia VF et al (2004) Bariatric surgery for severely overweight adolescents: concerns and recommendations. Pediatrics 114:217–223
33. Villareal DT, Apovian CM, Kushner RF, Klein S (2005) Obesity in older adults: technical review and position statement of the American Society for Nutrition and NAASO, The Obesity Society. Am J Clin Nutr 82:923–934
34. Busetto L, Romanato G, Zambon S et al (2009) The effects of weight changes after middle age on the rate of disability in an elderly population sample. J Am Geriatr Soc 57:1015–1021
35. Sugerman HJ, DeMaria EJ, Kellum JM et al (2004) Effects of bariatric surgery in older patients. Ann Surg 240:243–247
36. Quebbemann B, Engstrom D, Siegfried T et al (2005) Bariatric surgery in patients older than 65 years is safe and effective. Surg Obes Relat Dis 1:389–392
37. Hazzan D, Chin EH, Steinhagen E et al (2006) Laparoscopic bariatric surgery can be safe for treatment of morbid obesity in patients older than 60 years. Surg Obes Relat Dis 2:613–616
38. Taylor CJ, Layani L (2006) Laparoscopic adjustable gastric banding in patients > or =60 years old: is it worthwhile? Obes Surg 16:1579–1583
39. Dunkle-Blatter SE, St Jean MR, Whitehead C et al (2007) Outcomes among elderly bariatric patients at a high-volume center. Surg Obes Relat Dis 3:163–169
40. Busetto L, Angrisani L, Basso N et al (2008) Safety and efficacy of laparoscopic adjustable gastric banding in the elderly. Obesity 16:334–338

Bariatric Surgery Worldwide

3

Luigi Angrisani, Giampaolo Formisano, Antonella Santonicola,
Ariola Hasani, and Antonio Vitiello

3.1 Introduction

The obesity epidemic represents one of the main challenges for modern medicine. Data from the World Health Organization (WHO) estimates that more than 10% of the world's adult population is obese. Over the past decade, several studies have proved that bariatric surgery is the gold standard for the treatment of morbid obesity and weight-related comorbidities and is far more effective than nonsurgical interventions [1, 2]. However, only a small percentage of obese people actually undergo surgical treatment. Bariatric surgery has indeed evolved over time: several procedures have been developed over years, and some of them have already been abandoned. The choice of a specific bariatric procedure has been generally influenced by different factors, such as published results, worldwide trends, local conditions, and surgical-team experience. Four worldwide surveys of bariatric surgery have been published [3–6], which offer snapshots of the evolution of this discipline around the world. Recently, we reported an overview describing the number and types of procedures performed worldwide in 2013 [7], along with trends of the most common procedures over the 2003–2013 decade. Our analysis showed that Roux-en-Y gastric bypass (RYGB) was the most frequently performed procedure, sleeve gastrectomy (SG) experienced a steep increase (+37% from 2003 to 2013), while the popularity of adjustable gastric banding (AGB) significantly declined.

In 2014, the International Federation for the Surgery of Obesity and Metabolic Disorders (IFSO) endorsed a new survey, the aim of which was not only to update the previous study but to provide a comprehensive overview of

A. Santonicola (✉)
Gastrointestinal Unit, Department of Medicine and Surgery, University of Salerno
Salerno, Italy
e-mail: antonellasantonicola83@gmail.com

L. Angrisani (Ed), Bariatric and Metabolic Surgery,
Updates in Surgery
DOI: 10.1007/ 978-88-470-3944-5_3, © Springer-Verlag Italia 2017

the different endoluminal bariatric procedures performed worldwide. Herein we report the outcomes of our research.

3.2   Surgical and Endoluminal Procedures: Worldwide Data

Fifty-six of 60 (93.3%) IFSO bariatric societies contributed to the survey. The total number of bariatric/metabolic operations reported in 2014 was 593,792: surgical interventions were 97.6% (579,517), while only 2.4% (14,275) were endoluminal procedures. Numbers and percentages of the most common surgical procedures are listed in Table 3.1. Data regarding endoluminal treatment for morbid obesity are reported in Table 3.2.

Table 3.1 Number and percentage distribution of bariatric/metabolic surgical procedures

Surgical procedures	Number	Percentage
Sleeve gastrectomy (SG)	265,898	45.9
Roux-en-Y gastric bypass (RYGB)	229,455	39.6
Adjustable gastric banding (AGB)	42,388	7.4
Mini-gastric bypass/one anastomosis gastric bypass (MGB/OAGB)	10,403	1.8
Biliopancreatic diversion/duodenal switch (BPD-DS)	6,123	1.1
Miscellanea	25,250	4.3
Total	*579,517*	*100.0*

Table 3.2 Number and percentage distribution of endoluminal procedures

Endoscopic procedures	Number	Percentage
Orbera/BioEnterics intragastric balloon (BIB)	1,664	11.6
Obalon balloon	741	5.2
Spatz Adjustable Balloon System	62	0.4
Heliosphere Bag	7	0.05
Primary Obesity Surgery Endoluminal (POSE)	25	0.2
Apollo Overstitch Endosurgery	6	0.04
EndoBarrier	112	0.8
Not specified	11,658	81.6
Total	*14,275*	*100.0*

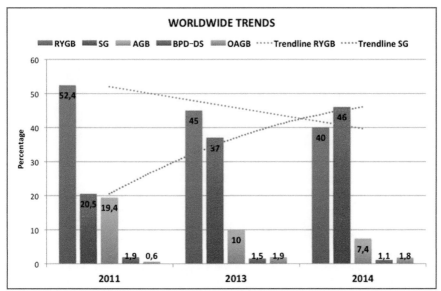

Fig. 3.1 Worldwide trend analysis. Data are reported in percentages. *Dotted line*: trendline for sleeve gastrectomy and Roux-en-Y gastric bypass. *RYGB* Roux-en-Y gastric bypass, *SG* sleeve gastrectomy, *AGB* adjustable gastric banding, *BPD-DS* biliopancreatic diversion/duodenal switch, *OAGB* one-anastomosis gastric bypass

3.3 Worldwide Trends

Comparison of data from the study with statistics from 2013 revealed that SG had the largest percentage increase among all surgical procedures, rocketing from 37% in 2013 to 45.9% in 2014, overcoming RYGB as the most performed bariatric surgery worldwide. On the other hand, RYGB and AGB had a percentage decrease of 5 and 2.6%, respectively. Mini-gastric bypass/one anastomosis gastric bypass (MGB/OAGB) and biliopancreatic diversion with duodenal switch (BPD-DS) plateaued. Short-term trends among main bariatric/metabolic surgical procedures (SG, RYGB, AGB, MGB/OAGB, and BPD-DS), expressed as relative proportion at fixed intervals (2011, 2013, 2014), are reported in Fig. 3.1.

3.4 Procedural Trends per Region

Regional changes from 2013 revealed a percentage increase (10.7–15.3%) of SG in USA/Canada, Europe, and Asia/Pacific. On the other hand, a percentage

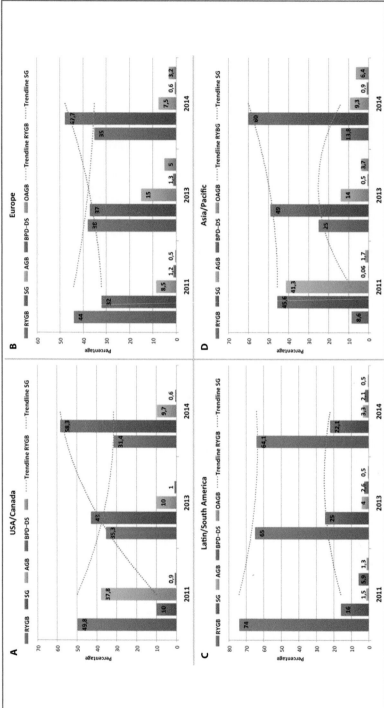

Fig. 3.2 Regional trend analysis. Data are reported in percentages. *Dotted line*: trendline for sleeve gastrectomy and Roux-en-Y gastric bypass. *A* USA/Canada, *B* Europe, *C* Latin/South America, *D* Asia/Pacific, *RYGB* Roux-en-Y gastric bypass, *SG* sleeve gastrectomy, *AGB* adjustable gastric banding, *BPD-DS* biliopancreatic diversion/duodenal switch, *OAGB* one-anastomosis gastric bypass

decrease of 3.9, 3, and 11% was observed for RYGB in USA/Canada, Europe, and Asia/Pacific, respectively. In Latin/South America, RYGB still represents the most popular procedure, while SG decreased by 2.9%. AGB plateaued in the American regions and declined in Europe and Asia/Pacific (–7.5 and –4.7%, respectively). BPD-DS plateaued in three of four IFSO chapters (USA/Canada, Asia/Pacific, Latin/South America), whereas a slight decrease was registered in Europe (–0.7%). MGB/OAGB increased in the Asia/Pacific region only (+2.7%); it plateaued in Latin/South America and slightly decreased in Europe (–0.7%). No data on MGB/OAGB were reported by USA/Canada. Data on regional trends are summarized in Fig. 3.2.

3.5   Discussion and Conclusions

Over recent years, different endoluminal procedures – Orbera intragastric balloon, BioEnterics intragastric balloon (BIB), Obalon balloon, Spatz Adjustable Balloon System, Heliosphere Bag, Primary Obesity Surgery Endoluminal (POSE) weight-loss procedure, StomaphyX, Apollo Overstitch Endosurgery, EndoBarrier – have gained popularity among bariatric surgeons in the attempt to fill the gap between medical and surgical treatment for borderline patients [8]. A total of 14,275 endoluminal procedures were reported in 2014, but since they have not been analyzed, it is not yet possible to determine a trend. However, they represent an evolving field of bariatric surgery, either as primary or revision procedures, and it is very likely that they will become more popular in the coming years; therefore, specific analysis is mandatory in future studies.

In order to optimize data collection, we added a specific section to the enquiry form of our previous survey [7], asking for endoscopic techniques. Moreover, we chose the definition "mini-gastric bypass/one anastomosis gastric bypass" (MGB/OAGB), as suggested by other authors [9, 10], in order to avoid data loss due to the high heterogeneity of definitions. This survey also provides short-term trend, from 2011 to 2014, of MGB/OAGB, the first experience on which was published by Rutledge in 2001 [11], and which then spread around the world, with some authors claiming to prove its efficacy and safety [12]. Worldwide, MGB/OAGB analysis reveals that this intervention increased only in Asia/Pacific and plateaued in all the other areas.

A 23.6% increase in bariatric/metabolic procedures was reported from 2013 to 2014, which may have been caused by the higher response rate (93.3 vs. 90.7%) compared with the previous survey [7]. Therefore, better reporting rather than a real increase may partially explain this result.

From 2003 to 2013, SG continuously gained success in all IFSO chapters, and in 2014, it was the most performed procedure globally, overcoming RYGB. As we hypothesized in our previous study [7], the easier surgical technique of SG compared with RYGB, together with the promising long-term outcomes [13,

14], could explain these findings. Analysis of regional trends shows that SG is the most common bariatric procedure in all regions except Latin/South America. In that area SG declined and RYGB remains the most performed intervention.

In conclusion, the current IFSO survey indicates that in 2014, there was a universal increase in bariatric surgery, and SG definitely replaced RYGB as the preferred intervention. Also bariatric endoluminal procedures have been reported consistently.

References

1. Picot J, Jones J, Colquitt JL et al (2009) The clinical effectiveness and cost-effectiveness of bariatric (weight loss) surgery for obesity: a systematic review and economic evaluation. Health Technol Assess 13:1–190, 215–357, iii-iv
2. Colquitt JL, Pickett K, Loveman E, Frampton GK (2014) Surgery for weight loss in adults. Cochrane Database Syst Rev 8:CD003641
3. Scopinaro N (1998) The IFSO and obesity surgery throughout the world. Obes Surg 8:3–8
4. Buchwald H, Williams SE (2004) Bariatric surgery worldwide 2003. Obes Surg 14:1157–1164
5. Buchwald H, Oien DM (2009) Metabolic/bariatric surgery worldwide 2008. Obes Surg 19:1605–1611
6. Buchwald H, Oien DM (2011) Metabolic/bariatric surgery worldwide. Obes Surg 23:427–436
7. Angrisani L, Santonicola A, Iovino P et al (2015) Bariatric surgery worldwide 2013. Obes Surg 25:1822–1832
8. Mathus-Vliegen EM (2014) Endoscopic treatment: the past, the present and the future. Best Pract Res Clin Gastroenterol 28:685–702
9. Rutledge R (2014) Naming the mini-gastric bypass. Obes Surg 24:2173
10. Carbajo MA, Luque-de-León E (2015) Mini-gastric bypass/one-anastomosis gastric bypass–standardizing the name. Obes Surg 25:858–859
11. Rutledge R (2001) The mini-gastric bypass: experience with the first 1,274 cases. Obes Surg 11:276–280
12. Georgiadou D, Sergentanis TN, Nixon A et al (2014) Efficacy and safety of laparoscopic mini gastric bypass. A systematic review. Surg Obes Relat Dis 10:984–991
13. Diamantis T, Apostolou KG, Alexandrou A et al (2014) Review of long-term weight loss results after laparoscopic sleeve gastrectomy. Surg Obes Relat Dis 10:177–183
14. Angrisani L, Santonicola A, Hasani A et al (2015) Five-year results of laparoscopic sleeve gastrectomy: effects on gastroesophageal reflux disease symptoms and co-morbidities. Surg Obes Relat Dis pii:S1550-7289(15)00855-2

Evolution of Bariatric Surgery in Italy: Results of the National Survey

4

Nicola Di Lorenzo, Giuseppe Navarra, Vincenzo Bruni, Ida Camperchioli, and Luigi Angrisani

4.1 Introduction

Over the last few decades, the number of overweight and obese individuals increased worldwide and became a major public health challenge in high-, middle-, and low-income countries. Overall, 31.8% of the Italian adult population – 39.8% men, 24.4% women – is overweight (body mass index, BMI $\geq$25 kg/m^2 and <30 kg/m^2) and 8.9% – 8.5% men, 9.4% women – is obese (BMI $\geq$30 kg/m^2) [1].

While governments, national health systems, and scientific societies draw strategies to battle the obesity epidemic, the disappointing long-term efficacy of conventional weight reduction treatments has contributed to the steep increase in the number of bariatric procedures performed worldwide [2–4]. Undoubtedly, bariatric surgery is the best available approach by which to achieve and maintain significant weight loss over the long term, together with a better quality of life, improvement in or remission of comorbidities, and a significant reduction in overall mortality [5–7]. Several surgical options are available: some have been proved to be safe and efficient; some are still investigational. The choice of a specific procedure depends on specific local conditions, such as a patient's alimentary disorders and comorbidities and the experience of surgical staff [8]. According to data from the annual survey of the International Federation for the Surgery of Obesity and Metabolic Disease (IFSO), the total number of metabolic/bariatric procedures performed worldwide progressed form 340,768 in 2011 to 468,609 in 2013 [8, 9].

In Italian hospitals belonging to the National Health system – as in some other countries aiming at zero mortality related to being overweight or obese [10] –

N. Di Lorenzo (✉)
Department of Experimental Medicine and Surgery, University of Rome Tor Vergata
Rome, Italy
e-mail: nicola.di.lorenzo@uniroma2.it

L. Angrisani (Ed), Bariatric and Metabolic Surgery,
Updates in Surgery
DOI: 10.1007/ 978-88-470-3944-5_4, © Springer-Verlag Italia 2017

bariatric surgery is indicated in patients with BMI >40 kg/m² or BMI >35 kg/m² with significant comorbidities in case of failure of nonsurgical treatments over an extended period, by previous psychological evaluation of the patient, and according to eligibility criteria established by the guidelines of the National Institutes of Health Consensus Development Conference Statement [11].

4.2   Creation and Evolution of the SICOB

The Italian Society for Obesity Surgery and Metabolic Diseases (SICOB) is a scientific community composed of Italian specialists battling obesity – including surgeons, psychologists and psychiatrists, nutritionists, and dietitians – with the purpose of improving the art and science of bariatric and metabolic surgery by continually increasing the quality and safety of care and treatment of obese people, providing educational and support programs for surgeons and integrated health professionals, and monitoring the number, type, safety, and long-term outcome of surgeries through the use of a national register.

The Society started its activity as the Italian Group of Bariatric Surgeons (GICO) in 1990 and became SICOB in 1995, with different targets [12]. Among them were to:

- promote and improve treatment of obesity and metabolic diseases through a multidisciplinary approach
- promote scientific research in this field
- regularly define and upgrade guidelines
- provide educational and support programs for surgeons and integrated health professionals
- become the recognized authority on bariatric and metabolic surgery
- monitor and certify number, type, safety, and long-term outcome of surgeries through the use of a national register
- serve professional needs of its members.

In the attempt to recognize the quality of treatment offered by bariatric centers in Italy, three levels of SICOB certified centers have been identified:

1. Excellence centers, which must perform at least four different surgical procedures recognized by SICOB, including redo surgery, with at least 100 surgical procedures/year.
2. Accredited centers, which must perform at least three different surgical procedures and no less than 50 surgical procedures/year.
3. Associated centers, which must perform at least two different surgical procedures with at least 25 surgical procedures/years.

All levels share the following features:
- they follow the same patient selection standards
- they have a multidisciplinary group
- they record all surgical activity on the national register

- they provide patient follow-up >50%, wholly recorded on the national register
- they have an available intensive care unit in the hospital.

4.3   Creation and Improvement of the SICOB Register

The SICOB register was created in January 1996 to record clinical data related to bariatric surgery in Italy [13].

The register holds data on the number of patients, is updated regularly, and allows a reliable comparison between surgical procedures using the same comparative method. Since 1996, three kinds of register have been designed:

The first (1996–2003) had 50 registry contributors and recorded 10,250 interventions (Table 4.1) that comprised: adjustable silicon gastric banding (ASGB) (43.3%), vertical banded gastroplasty (VBG) (33.2%), biliopancreatic diversion (BPD) (17%), Roux-en-Y gastric bypass (RYGB) (4.2%), BioEnterics intragastric balloon (BIB) (1.7%), nonadjustable gastric banding (NAGB) (0.5%), and other techniques (0.1%). In this first period, results in terms of percentage of excess weight loss (%EWL) at 5-year follow-up were 69.3% after BPD, 59.8% after VBG, and 39.9% after ASGB. There were early complications with 16.4% of RYGB, 10.6% of BPD, 8.2% of BIB, 7.8% of VBG, 2% of ASGB patients. Late complications with reinterventions occurred in 9.4% of ASGB (7% due to major complications), 5.3% of BPD, 3.4% of VBG, and 2.6% of RYGB procedures.

From 2004 to 2006, an online database was available, providing real-time updates, mandatory fields, avoidance of missing data, and improved data quality and processing efficiency. A total of 5975 surgical procedures were recorded on this database (Table 4.2): ASGB were performed in 57% of cases, RYGB in 21.5%, VBG in 9.7%, BPD in 7.3%, BIB in 2.6%, and sleeve gastrectomy (SG) in 1.9% of cases. Results in terms of %EWL at 5 years were 65% after BPD, 57.7% after RYGB, 57.3% after VBG, and 39.1% after ASGB; %EWL at 9-year follow-up were 66% after BPD, 55.2% after RYGB, 51.2% after ASGB, and 50.3% after VBG.

Table 4.1 Bariatric procedures recorded in Italy Between 1996 and 2003

Procedures	Number	Percentage
Adjustable silicon gastric banding (ASGB)	4437	43.3
Vertical banded gastroplasty (VBG)	3405	33.2
Biliopancreatic diversion (BPD)	1,741	17.0
Roux-en-Y gastric bypass (RYGB)	427	4.2
Bioenteric intragastric balloon (BIB)	175	1.7
Nonadjustable gastric banding (NAGB)	54	0.5
Others	11	0.1
Total	10,250	100.0

Table 4.2 Bariatric procedures recorded in Italy between 2004 and 2006

Procedures	Number	Percentage
Adjustable silicon gastric banding (ASGB)	3404	57.0
Roux-en-Y gastric bypass (RYGB)	1284	21.5
Vertical banded gastroplasty (VBG)	577	9.7
Biliopancreatic diversion (BPD)	439	7.3
BioEnterics intragastric balloon (BIB)	153	2.6
Sleeve gastrectomy (SG)	118	1.9
Total	*5975*	*100.0*

Table 4.3 Bariatric procedures performed in Italy between 2007 and 2010

Procedures	Number	Percentage
Adjustable silicon gastric banding (ASGB)	9384	46.2
Roux-en-Y gastric bypass (RYGB)	5125	25.2
Sleeve gastrectomy (SG)	3299	16.2
Biliopancreatic diversion (BPD) + duodenal switch (DS)	1529	7.5
Others	984	4.9
Total	*20,321*	*100.0*

Table 4.4 Bariatric procedures performed in Italy between 2011 and 2015

Procedures	Number	Percentage
Sleeve gastrectomy (SG)	16,805	38.9
Adjustable silicon gastric banding (ASGB)	12,050	27.9
Roux-en-Y gastric bypass (RYGB)	8734	20.2
Mini-gastric bypass	2477	5.7
Biliopancreatic diversion (BPD) + duodenal switch	1162	2.7
Others	1048	2.4
Gastric plication	911	2.2
Total	*43,187*	*100.0*

A newly designed database was finally implemented in 2007 to increase the amount of data entry on follow-up, and from then to the end of 2015, 63,508 bariatric and metabolic surgical procedures were recorded on the register (Tables 4.3 and 4.4): ASGB in 33.7% of cases, SG in 31.6%, RYGB in 21.8%, BPD and duodenal switch in 4.2%, mini-gastric bypass in 3.9%, gastric plication in 1.6%, and other procedures in 3.2%.

As is clearly shown by collected data, the key objective of the national register – to accumulate sufficient data to allow a comprehensive report on outcomes following bariatric surgery – has been met. Over the last few years, more procedures have been recorded, new centers have begun uploading their caseloads, and long-term follow-up data are available for more patients. At present, the register allows constant monitoring of bariatric surgery in Italy, not just in terms of number of procedures performed but especially in terms of outcomes. It renders SICOB, de facto, the recognized authority on bariatric surgery, since it is the only scientific body in Italy to contain data not only on the safety but also on long-term outcomes, such as %EWL and comorbidity remission.

4.4   Results of the National Survey

Thanks to data extracted from the national register, SICOB recently released data of a national survey on bariatric surgery in Italy [14]. From 1996 to the present, SICOB centers grew from 53 to 108: 56 centers (51.9%) are in the north, 24 (22.2%) in the center, 21 (19.4%) in the south, and 7 (6.5%) on the islands. Excellence centers have grown from 28% in 2011 to 37% in 2015, while centers performing <50 procedures decreased from 48% to 33%. Bariatric surgeries performed have increased from 5974 procedures in 2008 to 11,435 in 2015, with >95% of the them being performed laparoscopically over the last five years. Data on type of surgery performed between 2008 and 2015 show a clear drop in bands, down from >50% to 21%; a limited decrease in gastric bypass, down to 16.6% from 23.6%, which is compensated by the number of mini-gastric bypasses performed in 2015 (870; 7.6% of cases). During the same period, the most striking data is the explosion of sleeve gastrectomies performed, jumping from 8.9% to 48.5% of cases.

The reason for these changes could be related to suboptimal long-term results after gastric bandings and a limited but still present number of cases of weight regain. At present, sleeve gastrectomy is by far the most popular procedure because it is quick, efficient, and can be converted to duodenal switch (DS) or RYGB in case of weight regain.

References

1. Gallus S, Odone A, Lugo A et al (2013) Overweight and obesity prevalence and determinants in Italy: an update to 2010. Eur J Nutr 52:677–685
2. Lecube A, de Hollanda A, Calañas A et al (2015) Trends in bariatric surgery in Spain in the twenty-first century: baseline results and 1-month follow-up of the RICIBA, a national registry. Obes Surg [Epub ahead of print] doi:10.1007/s11695-015-2001-3

3. Neira M, de Onis M (2006) The Spanish strategy for nutrition, physical activity and the prevention of obesity. Br J Nutr 96(Suppl 1):S8–S11
4. Buchwald H, Oien DM (2008) Metabolic/bariatric surgery worldwide. Obes Surg 19:1605–1611
5. Courcoulas AP, Christian NJ, Belle SH et al (2013) Weight change and health outcomes at 3 years after bariatric surgery among individuals with severe obesity. JAMA 310:2416–2425
6. Buchwald H, Avidor Y, Braunwald E et al (2004) Bariatric surgery: a systematic review and meta-analysis. JAMA 92:1724–1737
7. Ramos-Levi AM, Rubio Herrera MA (2014) Metabolic surgery: quo vadis? Endocrinol Nutr 61:35–46
8. Angrisani L, Santonicola A, Iovino P et al (2015) Bariatric surgery worldwide 2013. Obes Surg 25:1822–1832
9. Buchwald H, Oien DM (2011) Metabolic/bariatric surgery worldwide. Obes Surg 23:427–436
10. Fort JM, Vilallonga R, Lecube A et al (2013) Bariatric surgery outcomes in a European Centre of Excellence (CoE). Obes Surg 23:1324–1332
11. NIH Consensus Development Conferences (1992) Gastrointestinal surgery for severe obesity: National Institutes of Health Consensus Development Conference Statement. Am J Clin Nutr 55(2 Suppl):615S–619S
12. SICOB (2016) Società Italiana di Chirurgia dell'Obesità e delle Malattie Metaboliche http://www.sicob.org
13. Toppino M e partecipanti Registro SICOB(2004) Il registro SICOB. In: Chirurgia bariatrica. Chap 30, pp 231–233. http://editoria.sichirurgia.info/sic/pdf/editoria/RelazioniBiennali/Basso/30.pdf
14. SICOB - Italian Society of Bariatric and Metabolic Surgery (2016) Indagine conoscitiva: Anno 2015. www.sicob.org/area_04_medici/00_indagine.aspx

Gastric Banding

5

Maurizio De Luca, Gianni Segato, David Ashton, Cesare Lunardi, and Franco Favretti

5.1 Introduction

Despite major changes in bariatric surgery, laparoscopic adjustable gastric banding (LAGB) remains a popular and effective surgical option for managing obesity and related metabolic disease. A major reason for its popularity is that it is the least invasive of all surgical interventions currently available. LAGB was the first bariatric operation to be performed laparoscopically and marked a major transition from the much more aggressive laparotomic era to the minimally invasive laparoscopic era. Since 1993, LAGB has evolved into a routine laparoscopic procedure, and nowadays, most band implants are performed as day cases. LAGB is a remarkably safe operation from both a general surgical and a bariatric perspective. It facilitates short-term hospitalization and has very low rates of early and late complications, which are also less severe than those associated with other, more invasive, procedures. Moreover, because LAGB is a nonmutilating procedure and does not require removal of tissue or any alteration of gastric or intestinal continuity, it is easily reversed. In some bariatric centers, LAGB is now performed via a single umbilical incision.

Despite its popularity among patients and its minimal invasiveness, LAGB is a demanding procedure that should not be performed on an occasional basis in medical facilities with little experience in the postoperative management of the gastric band patient. Successful long–term outcomes after LAGB depend on a number of variables, including surgical technique and skills, careful patient selection, managing patient expectations, and close postoperative monitoring and follow-up. The latter should include expert band adjustment, early intervention for any band-related problems, and intensive behavioral support to maintain appropriate lifestyle modification. Safe and successful band adjustment require

M. De Luca (✉)
Department of Surgery, Montebelluna Treviso Hospital
Montebelluna, Italy
e-mail: nnwdel@tin.it

L. Angrisani (Ed), Bariatric and Metabolic Surgery,
Updates in Surgery
DOI: 10.1007/ 978-88-470-3944-5_5, © Springer-Verlag Italia 2017

knowledge of the band's physical specifications and compliance with a detailed adjustment protocol [1–4]. It is also important to consider the physiological behavior of the implanted gastric band, particularly during swallowing and gastric-pouch emptying. Activating the satiety mechanism requires patient understanding of the importance of eating slowly and an awareness of when to stop eating. Patients should be trained to eat only when they are hungry and to eat until they are not hungry – not until they are full. Behavioral compliance includes choosing foods of the right texture and a good balance of macronutrients, as well as avoiding energy-dense snacks. Attention to all these elements of care is essential if suboptimal results are to be avoided [4, 5].

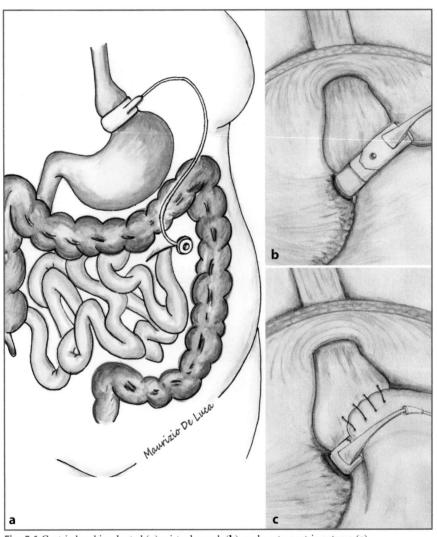

Fig. 5.1 Gastric band implanted (**a**), virtual pouch (**b**), and gastrogastric sutures (**c**)

5.2 Surgical Technique

5.2.1 Preparation for Surgery

Hematological and biochemical tests may include a full blood count (in particular, to identify polycythemia), serum electrolytes, blood glucose response curve to determine glycemic index, kidney and liver function tests, and blood coagulation tests. If the patient's history shows evidence of thyroid and/or adrenal gland dysfunction, a targeted hormonal study should be considered. In some centers, routine preoperative tests also include echocardiogram, chest radiography, liver ultrasound, esophagogastroduodenoscopy (EGDS), and spirometry.

5.2.1.1 Patient and Surgical Team Positioning

When using the 30° reverse Trendelenburg position, the first surgeon is positioned between the patient's legs and the second surgeon on the patient's right or left side.

5.2.1.2 Procedural Steps

The procedure's key points, as defined and standardized at the beginning of the LAGB experience (1993–1995) are to identify the reference points for dissection (most surgeons take this to be the equator of the balloon of a calibration tube containing 25 mL of air) and the left diaphragmatic pillar. A retrogastric tunnel is created above the peritoneal reflection of the lesser sac, a "virtual" pouch is created, and retention sutures are placed to avoid slippage (Figs. 5.1 and 5.2).

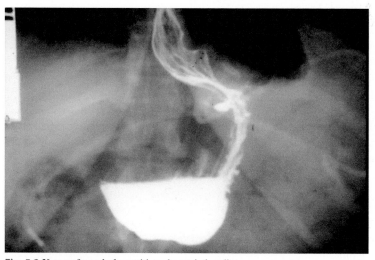

Fig. 5.2 X-ray of regularly positioned gastric banding

5.2.1.3 Reference Points

Dissection on the lesser curvature is made on the equator of the balloon of the calibration tube inserted through the mouth, although some surgeons no longer use the calibration tube. On the greater curvature, the reference point is the angle of His. Identifying these two reference points is essential for correct band positioning.

5.2.2 Perigastric Technique

Dissection is made 2 cm below the cardia on the lesser curvature, as close as possible to the gastric wall, taking care not to damage it and to preserve Latarjet's nerve. Under direct vision, a small, narrow passage is created, clearly identifying and preserving the stomach's posterior wall. Retrogastric dissection, which is meant to connect the two previously identified reference points, must be carried out above the peritoneal reflection of the lesser sac. The gastric band and its connecting tube are introduced into the abdominal cavity through the trocar of the left hypochondrium and then locked. In order to introduce the gastric band into the abdominal cavity, a 15- or 18-mm-diameter trocar may not be required. Instead, some surgeons simply remove the 10-mm trocar from the left hypochondrium and then bluntly insert the band following its route through the abdominal wall. Three to five, gastrogastric sutures are placed between the seromuscular layers of the anterior wall of the stomach proximally and then distally to the band. These sutures prevent stomach slippage above the band. Thus, a "virtual" proximal gastric pouch is created. Instead of individual stitches, some surgeons apply a running suture, some add a single gastropexy stitch, and others do not use sutures of any kind. The connection tube is then retracted through the port in the left hypochondrium. The access port is secured with sutures (or with a polypropylene mesh) to the fascia of the anterior abdominal wall in the left hypochondrium. Band adjustments can then be made through the access port using 0.9% saline. By altering the diameter of the band stoma in this way, a satiety response can be created.

The first band adjustment is usually carried out some 5–8 weeks after surgery. Thereafter, adjustments are calibrated against the patient's weight loss. Most centers no longer use radiological imaging for routine band adjustments, but it may be required in circumstances in which the port is difficult to access or where other problems, such as slippage, may be suspected.

5.2.3 Pars Flaccida Technique

In the last 15 years, this approach has been proposed for creating the retrogastric tunnel. The technique has rapidly gained consensus and is widely used, as it is considered easier to learn and probably less susceptible to complications (perforations and slippage). Once the lesser pars flaccida of the lesser omentum has been divided up to the extragastric vagal fibers (which should be preserved), the caudate lobe of the liver and the right diaphragmatic pillar become visible. This is the starting point for the blunt dissection toward the angle of His, remaining in front of the plane of the diaphragmatic pillars, exactly as in fundoplication procedures for gastroesophageal reflux disease or hiatal hernia repair. Introduction and positioning of the band, band locking, sutures, port positioning, and band adjustment is the same as in the perigastric technique.

5.2.4   Pars Flaccida versus Perigastric Technique

It is possible to use a combination of the two previous techniques, especially in the case of visceral obesity, to avoid too much tissue being included in the band and consequent risk of early gastric stenosis. The dissection starts according to the pars flaccida approach and, once the tunnel is created, shifts to the perigastric technique. An anteroposterior perigastric opening along the lesser curvature is created close the equator of the calibration tube balloon, and the tip of the calibration tube is then grasped and pulled through. Therefore, the band is positioned from the angle of His to the perigastric window. Band introduction, positioning, and locking; sutures; port positioning; and band adjustment are the same than in perigastric technique [6].

5.3   Results

5.3.1   Weight Loss

In their systematic review, Buchwald et al. found a mean percentage of excess weight loss (%EWL) of 47.5% for patients who underwent bariatric surgery [7]. Tice et al. reported 48% EWL at 1 year [8]. A recent report on a large series of gastric bands from the UK [9] reported results on 2356 primary gastric band procedures. Mean excess body mass index (BMI) loss at 1, 2, 3, and 5 years was $43.97 \pm 27.4\%$, $51.8 \pm 37.41\%$, $49.7 \pm 36.88\%$, and $52.6 \pm 41.74\%$, respectively [9].

Several studies have compared weight loss between the gastric band and Roux-en-Y gastric bypass (RYGB), and results suggest that although after RYGB initial weight loss was greater, after 2–5 years there was no significant difference in %EWL. These finding are consistent with a systematic review by O'Brien et al., who found that mean %EWL for standard gastric bypass was higher than for gastric banding at year 1 and 2 but was not statistically different at years 3–7. Note that this was primarily attributed to fading of the effect of RYGB, whereas weight loss with the band remains relatively stable [10].

5.3.2 Type 2 Diabetes Mellitus

Buchwald et al. described a gradation of effects for diabetes resolution following different surgical techniques. Regarding gastric banding, their systematic review reported 56.7% of patients achieving diabetes resolution and 80% achieving resolution or improvement [11].

5.3.3 Mortality

In the Swedish Obese Subject (SOS) Study, the adjusted 10-year mortality rate was significantly (31%) lower than in the nonsurgical group, and most surgical patients were treated with gastric banding. A study comparing LAGB versus nonsurgical treatment showed a statistically significant 60% reduction in total mortality in favor of the LAGB group at a mean follow-up of 5.7 and 7.2 years, respectively [12]. In addition, Peeters et al. compared the mortality rate in 1468 morbidly obese patients treated by gastric banding with 5960 patients from an established population-based control group. They found that the surgically treated group were 73% less likely to die of their disease than those in the control group [13].

5.4   Complications (According to Clavien-Dindo Classification)

LAGB surgery is not without complications, but these occur on a smaller scale and have a much lower risk profile compared with other methods currently used in obesity surgery [14, 15].

5.4.1   Gastric Perforation (Grade IIIb)

The stomach may be perforated during surgery (0.2–0.8% of cases), mainly during creation of the retrogastric tunnel. This step can be difficult in patients with very high BMI, visceral obesity, and in men. Gastric perforation is characterized by free leakage of gastric contents into the peritoneum. Confirmation is provided by a methylene blue test. If the perforation is detected during surgery, and if it occurs in a site distant from the band, some surgeons have repaired the stomach laparoscopically and placed the band successfully. If exposure is not satisfactory, it is advisable to postpone band placement, suture the stomach wall, drain the area, and place a nasogastric tube in situ. If the perforation is detected postoperatively and gross contamination has already occurred, causing peritonitis, the band must be removed, the gastric wall (possibly) sutured, and drainage performed with a nasogastric tube.

5.4.2 Stomach Slippage (Grade I if Band Deflation, Grade IIIb if Band Removal or Repositioning)

Stomach slippage (1.0–5.0%) is the postoperative development of a large upper gastric pouch. Often referred to a gastric prolapse and often confused with pouch dilatation, this complication can occur anteriorly and/or posteriorly. It can be caused by inadequate surgical technique (reduced incidence with pars flaccid) or lack of compliance on the part of the patient, especially overeating in the presence of a tight band. An upper gastrointestinal (GI) X-ray series is diagnostic. Treatment consists of simple band deflation (90% of cases) or surgical removal and/or repositioning of the band (10% of cases).

5.4.3 Stoma Obstruction (Grade I if Band Deflation, Grade IIIb if Band Removal or Repositioning)

Stoma obstruction (1.5%) is defined as an obstruction to the passage of food from the gastric pouch to the rest of the stomach. It can happen early or late in the postoperative period. Early causes are a small band applied over a thick gastroesophageal junction (GEJ) or too distal from the GEJ, too much tissue inside the band, postoperative edema of the area incorporated by the band due to hematoma, or postoperative reaction. Late stoma obstructions are usually related to gastric pouch dilatation, stomach slippage, erosion, pouchitis, and/or esophagitis caused by poor eating habits. An upper GI X-ray series is diagnostic. Treatment consists of simple band deflation (80%) or surgical ban removal/repositioning (20%).

5.4.4 Oesophageal and Gastric Pouch Dilatation (Grade I if Band Deflation, Grade IIIb if Band Removal or Repositioning)

Oesophageal and gastric pouch dilatation (4%) without stomach slippage is caused by band overinflation resulting in mechanically severe outlet obstruction, creation of an oversized pouch during surgery (band placed too low or malpositioned), patient's lack of compliance regarding oral intake (inappropriate food intake, insufficient chewing of food, overeating causing vomiting). An upper GI X-ray series is diagnostic. Treatment consists of simple band deflation (95%) or surgical band removal/repositioning (5%).

5.4.5 Erosion (Grade IIIb for Band Removal by Laparoscopy or Endoscopy)

Band erosion (0.8%) is defined as partial or complete band migration into the gastric lumen of the stomach. This complication renders the band ineffective in terms of weight loss and always requires band removal. Causes of erosion can be a combination of small, undetected injuries to the gastric wall during surgery; necrosis due to pressure of the band; and access port infection. Some authors believe that first the access port becomes infected and the infection then travels along the tubing to the band, causing erosion. However, most surgeons believe that access port infection is almost always a late manifestation of erosion. An upper GI X-ray series and consequent esophagogastric devascularization and splenectomy (EGDS) are diagnostic. Treatment consists of band removal (5%) via laparoscopy or orally by endoscopy, especially if the band is contained completely within the gastric lumen. If endoscopic removal is contemplated, general anesthesia is strongly recommended [16, 17].

5.4.6   Gastric Necrosis (Grade IVa)

Gastric necrosis (0.1%) means necrosis of the upper gastric pouch and may occur early in the postoperative period or later, when it is likely to be the result of a long-term undetected stomach slippage/pouch dilatation, both of which increase pressure on the gastric wall, thereby decreasing blood supply to the fundus. The theoretical link between stomach slippage and necrosis is precisely why stomach slippage must be considered a surgical emergency. An upper GI X-ray series and consequent EGDS are diagnostic.

Treating gastric necrosis consists of exploratory laparoscopy or laparotomy, the methylene blue test, gastric suture, gastric resection, or nasogastric tube and drainage.

5.4.7   Tubing/Port Access System (Grade IIIa)

The port is an essential component of the band system, and its placement requires careful attention. The tubing/port access system can be linked to design features at the interface between the access port and the tubing and in part to the method of port placement. Port inversion (flipped port) and leakage are the most frequent problems. Treatment consists of port repositioning or replacement, and in most cases, surgery can be performed under local anaesthesia (3%).

Widely differing complication rates are reported in the literature [18]. This is likely to be partly attributable to the surgical technique deployed, but primarily to the quality of the after-care and follow-up.

5.5   Conclusions

Whereas further refinement of surgical technique may reduce complication rates, it is unlikely to improve the 50–60% EWL rate, which is such a consistent feature of the majority of long-term LAGB studies. In order to achieve better long-term results with the band, it is necessary to focus greater effort toward a better understanding of what should be regarded as best practice regarding long-term follow-up and behavioral support. We know that the magnitude of early postoperative weight loss predicts long-term outcomes, but beyond this observation, little is known. It is a remarkable fact that even after tens of thousands of gastric bands have been implanted over the last 15 years, there is still no consensus regarding the postoperative optimal adjustment algorithm, nutritional management, or physical activity. During the next decade, we must move away from observational studies with descriptive statistics to a much greater emphasis on hypothesis testing within the context of large-scale randomized trials.

References

1. Cadiere GB, Bruyns J, Himpens J et al (1994) Laparoscopic gastroplasty for morbid obesity. Br J Surg 81:1524–1525
2. Dixon JB, Dixon ME, O'Brien PE (2001) Pre-operative predictors of weight loss at 1-year after LAP-BAND surgery. Obes Surg 11:200–207
3. Favretti F, Cadiere GB, Segato G et al (1995) Laparoscopic adjustable gastric banding (LAP-BAND): technique and results. Obes Surg 364–371
4. Favretti F, Ashton D, Busetto L et al (2009) The gastric banding: first-choice procedure for obesity surgery. World J Surg 33:2039–2048
5. Busetto L, Segato G, De Marchi F et al (2002) Outcome predictors in morbidly obese recipients of an adjustable gastric band. Obes Surg 12:83–92
6. Di Lorenzo N, Furbetta F, Favretti F et al (2010) Laparoscopic adjustable gastric banding via pars flaccida versus perigastric positioning: technique, complications, and results in 2,549 patients. Surg Endosc 24:1519–1523
7. Buchwald H, Oien DM (2011) Metabolic/bariatric surgery worldwide. Obes Surg 23:427–436
8. Tice JA, Karliner L, Walsh J (2008) Gastric banding or bypass? A systematic review comparing the two most popular bariatric procedures. Am J Med 121:885–893
9. Puzziferri N, Roshek TB 3rd, Mayo HG (2014) Long-term follow-up after bariatric surgery: a systematic review. JAMA 312: 934–942
10. O'Brien PE, Brown WA, Dixon JB (2005) Obesity, weight loss and bariatric surgery. Med J Aust 183:310–314
11. Buchwald H, Estok R, Fahrbach K (2009) Weight and type 2 diabetes after bariatric surgery: systematic review and meta-analysis. Am J Med 122:248–256
12. Sjöström L (2008) Bariatric surgery and reduction in morbidity and mortality: experience from SOS study. Int J Obes (Lond) 32(Suppl 7):S93–S97
13. Peeters A, O'Brien PE, Laurie C, Anderson M (2007) Substantial intentional weight loss and mortality in severely obese. Ann Surg 246:1028–1033
14. De Luca M, Busetto L, Segato G et al (2011) Laparoscopic adjustable gastric banding (LAP-BAND): diagnosis, prevention and treatment of complications. In: Hakim N, Favretti F, Segato G, Dillemans B (eds) Bariatric surgery. Imperial College Press, World Scientific, London, pp 125–152
15. Favretti F, Segato G, De Luca M, Busetto L (2007) Minimally invasive bariatric surgery. Laparoscopic adjustable gastric banding: revisional surgery. Springer, New York, pp 213–230
16. Di Lorenzo N, Lorenzo M, Furbetta F et al (2013) Intragastric gastric band migration: erosion – an analysis of multicenter experience on 177 patients. Surg Endosc 27:1151–1157

17. De Jong IC, Tan KG, Oostenbroek RJ (2000) Adjustable silicone gastric banding: a series with three cases of band erosion. Obes Surg 10:26–32

18. Fabry H, Van Hee R, Hendrickx L, Totté E (2002) A technique for prevention of port complications after laparoscopic adjustable silicone gastric banding. Obes Surg 12:285–288

Sleeve Gastrectomy

6

Emanuele Soricelli, Giovanni Casella, Alfredo Genco,
and Nicola Basso

6.1   Introduction

Sleeve gastrectomy (SG) was performed for the first time in 1988 by Hess and Hess as part of a hybrid malabsorptive procedure, the biliopancreatic diversion with duodenal switch (BPD-DS) [1]. Unlike the original Scopinaro biliopancreatic diversion (BPD), which consisted of a horizontal subtotal gastrectomy with a gastroileal anastomosis, the BPD-DS combined a vertical gastrectomy, namely SG, with an end-to-end suprapapillary duodenoileal anastomosis. The rational was to maintain a proper gastric restriction, avoiding the occurrence of marginal ulcers at the gastroileal anastomosis, the incidence of which was considerably high after BPD [2].

Several studies show that BPD-DS was as effective as the Scopinaro BPD in terms of weight loss, moreover, the malabsorption-related side-effects, such as diarrhea, number of daily stools, vomiting, bone pain, and lack of serum vitamins and minerals, were less severe after BPD-DS than after BPD because of the longest common channel's length in the former (100 cm vs. 50 cm, respectively) [3]. In 2000, Ren et al. demonstrated the feasibility of BPD-DS with a laparoscopic approach [4]; however, in high-risk, superobese patients, it was affected by a high incidence of complications and mortality. In order to reduce the overall surgical risk, Regan et al. proposed splitting the procedure into two surgical stages: laparoscopic SG (LSG) in the first stage, and BPD-DS after an average 11-month interval [5].

The good results of LSG, as a first stage, in terms of weight loss and resolution of comorbidities and the great compliance of patients, encouraged spreading of this procedure. Moreover, a mounting number of published studies supported the effectiveness of LSG as a sole operation [6]. As a consequence,

E. Soricelli (✉)
Department of Surgical Sciences, Sapienza University of Rome
Rome, Italy
e-mail: emanuele.soricelli@uniroma1.it

L. Angrisani (Ed), Bariatric and Metabolic Surgery,
Updates in Surgery
DOI: 10.1007/ 978-88-470-3944-5_6, © Springer-Verlag Italia 2017

in 2009, the American Society for Metabolic and Bariatric Surgery (ASMBS) issued a position statement recommending LSG as an approved primary bariatric procedure [7].

At first, LSG was classified as a restrictive procedure, since its weight-loss effectiveness was entirely attributed to reduction of the gastric capacity. However, it soon became evident that significant modifications of gastrointestinal hormones play a preeminent role. Changes in ghrelin (GHR), glucagon-like peptide-1 (GLP-1), and peptide tyrosine-tyrosine (PYY), induced by the gastric resection, are of paramount importance in weight loss and glucose homeostasis effects of the procedure [8].

At present LSG is the second most performed bariatric procedure after Roux-en-Y gastric bypass (RYGB), and it has the fastest increment rate in the last decade [9]. The common perception of LSG as a safe and easy-to-perform procedure has had a major role in its noteworthy worldwide spread. Because of the lack of gastrointestinal anastomosis and the short operative time, many surgeons consider LSG an ideal option to start a novel bariatric activity. This might represent a boomerang effect, because LSG entails some key technical points that require adequate training: dissection of the stomach from the spleen, and complete detachment of the posterior gastric wall from the anterior aspect of the pancreas and diaphragmatic crura are necessary to perform an adequate fundectomy, which is of utmost importance for both the restrictive and the hormonal effects of LSG. Furthermore, the postoperative course can be affected by life-threatening complications such as gastric leak, the management of which requires a specific experience and should be performed in dedicated institutions.

6.2   Surgical Technique

The laparoscopic technique was standardized by Ren et al. in 2000 [4]. However, during the following years, several details have been modified. In this chapter, we emphasize technical points in light of our own experience of ~900 cases since 2002.

6.2.1   Preparation for Surgery

In all patients, preoperative workup included history and physical examination, routine laboratory tests, esophagogastroduodenoscopy, abdominal ultrasonography, nutritional and psychiatric evaluation, and additional examinations and/or consultations when indicated. The day before surgery, subcutaneous low-molecular-weight heparin (LMWH) is administered.

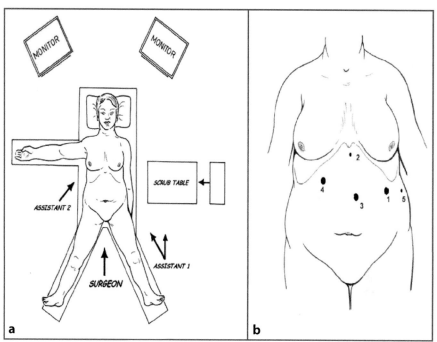

Fig. 6.1 a Operating room setup. **b** Trocar placement scheme. *1* left subcostal, *2* subxyphoid, *3* optical, *4* right subcostal, *5* left anterior axillary line

6.2.2 Patient and Surgical Team Positioning

The patient is positioned in a 30° reverse Trendelenburg position with legs abducted. The surgeon stands between the patient's legs while the first assistant, holding the camera, is on the left side of the patient, beside the scrub nurse (Fig. 6.1a). A second assistant is placed on the right side. Five trocars (four 12-mm and one 5-mm) are placed in the upper abdominal quadrants, as described in Fig. 6.1b.

6.2.3 Procedure Step by Step

- Identification of the pylorus: Using a marked grasper and stretching the gastric wall, a distance of 4–6 cm along the greater gastric curvature is measured and marked. Some authors suggest 2–3 cm as the distance from the pylorus as where to begin the gastric resection. However, antrum resection may result in a defective pumping mechanism, causing nausea to the patient because of delayed gastric emptying.

- Skeletonization of the greater curvature: By means of radiofrequency or ultrasound energy devices, the gastrocolic ligament is dissected close to the gastric wall starting at the median third of the greater curvature, where the ligament is thin. The dissection proceeds downward to the antrum until the 4- to 6-cm mark is reached. In this area, access to the omental bursa might be difficult because of the frequent presence of adhesions between the posterior wall of the stomach and the anterior aspect of the pancreas. Then, skeletonization proceeds upward to the angle of His. Attachments with the upper pole of the spleen should be divided carefully in order to avoid splenic injury or bleeding from short gastric vessels.
- Complete mobilization of the fundus and posterior gastric wall: In this phase, the surgeon can move his or her left hand from the right subcostal trocar to the subxiphoid trocar to facilitate the approach to the gastroesophageal area. The dissection of the fundus is completed when clear exposure of the left diaphragmatic pillar is obtained (Fig. 6.2a). If the Belsey's fat pad on the anterior aspect of the gastroesophageal junction is redundant, its resection may be useful to properly expose the area where the stapler will be placed. The posterior gastric wall must be completely freed from adhesions. When present, posterior gastric vessels should be divided, as they can lessen compliance of the stomach during resection. At the end of mobilization, the left gastric vessels and left crus are clearly exposed, and the stomach can be easily moved on this axis – like the page of a book (Fig. 6.2b). The proper accomplishment of these surgical steps is of primary importance in order to achieve a complete fundectomy. Since GHR secretion is predominant in the gastric fundus, its ablation plays a main role in the LSG mechanism of action [10, 11]. On the other hand, accurate mobilization of the gastric fundus and gastroesophageal junction entails the division of the short gastric vessels and, when present, the posterior gastric artery and phrenic branches [12]. This might hamper the blood supply in this area, favoring the onset of gastric leaks, which occur quite uniformly at the uppermost part of the suture line. During this surgical step, risks (leak) and benefits (functional result) should be carefully weighted.
- Inspection of the hiatal area and possible hiatoplasty: Enlarged hiatus and hiatal hernias must be identified. A hiatal orifice with a diameter >3 cm is considered abnormal (Fig. 6.2c). A macroscopically evident fingerprint indentation of the diaphragm just above the esophageal emergence should be considered suspicious for the presence of a hiatal hernia, indicating dissection of the hiatal area. This can be easily approached from the left, as the fundus has been previously mobilized. When present, the hernia sac and gastroesophageal fat pad are dissected and reduced within the abdominal cavity. A posterior hiatoplasty is performed by approaching the right and the left diaphragmatic pillars with two or three interrupted nonabsorbable sutures (Fig. 6.2d).

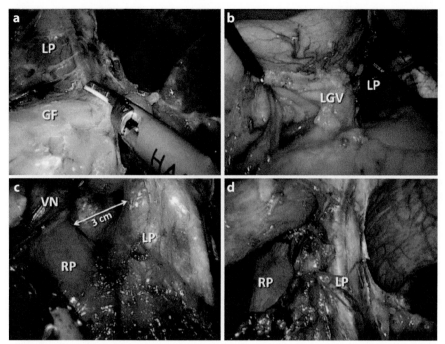

Fig. 6.2 a Dissection of the gastric fundus from the anterior aspect of the left pillar. **b** Left gastric vessels are visualized together with the left pillar. **c** Enlarged hiatus. **d** Posterior hiatoplasty with nonabsorbable stitches. *LP* left pillar, *GF* gastric fundus, *LGV* left gastric vessels, *VN* vagus nerve, *RP* right pillar

- Orogastric tube insertion: This tube is inserted by the anesthesiologist and pushed down, possibly through the pylorus. It is then placed against the lesser curvature in order to calibrate the resection. In our clinical practice, we use a 48-Fr bougie, although in the literature the use of tube sizes from 30- to 60-Fr is reported [13]. Literature data correlate the smaller size of the bougie to a higher incidence of gastric leaks. Furthermore, a clear relationship between bougie size and postoperative weight loss is lacking [14–18]. In our experience, the residual capacity of the gastric remnant does not depend on bougie size but mainly on the degree of countertraction exerted on the stomach walls when resecting and on accurate dissection of the gastric fundus [19].
- Gastric resection and staple-line reinforcement: This step is performed using a linear stapler applied alongside the calibrating bougie. The height of the cartridges must be chosen according to gastric-wall thickness, since it decreases from the antrum to the corpus and fundus. We prefer a staple height of 4.4 or 4.1 mm near the antrum and 3.8 or 3.5 mm on the corpus and fundus. In revision surgery cases, the use of higher staples might be advisable because of the presence of thick scar tissue. Before closing and

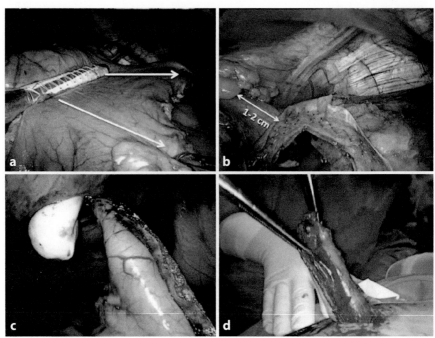

Fig. 6.3 a Homogeneous countertraction of both anterior and posterior gastric walls by means of two graspers placed exactly at the greater curvature. **b** The last staple is fired 1–2 cm from the angle of His. **c** The caudal tip of the resected stomach is extracted, using a grasper, through the slightly enlarged right subcostal access. **d** Careful extraction of the specimen without retrieval bags or endoloop

firing the stapler, the anterior and posterior gastric walls should be stretched homogeneously by two graspers placed exactly at the greater curve (Fig. 6.3a). At the incisura angularis, stretching is somewhat loosened to avoid functional strictures. The last cartridge is fired 1–2 cm away from the angle of His (Fig. 6.3b) so that the staple line does not fall within the critical area [12]. The staple line is reinforced by buttressing with absorbable polymer membrane (Seamguard, Gore) and meticulously checked for bleeding spots, which can be managed by using hemostatic clips or stitches. After moving the stomach specimen away from the left subcostal space, the final end of the membrane is fixed with two nonabsorbable sutures to the left pillar to avoid sliding of the stomach tubule into the mediastinum (Fig. 6.4b). A nasogastric tube is positioned in the gastric remnant, and a methylene blue dye test is routinely performed to check for complete sealing of the staple line and to evaluate the residual gastric capacity, usually 60–80 mL.

- Specimen extraction: The specimen is extracted by grabbing its distal end with a grasper. It is easily brought out of the abdominal cavity through the slightly enlarged right subcostal access. Care must be taken not to open the specimen during these manoeuvres (Fig. 6.3c, d). No retrieval bags or endoloops are needed [20]. A gauze soaked in povidone-iodine solution (betadine) is left for 1–2 min at the retrieval site to avoid wound infection. Drains are not routinely placed, and the nasogastric tube is removed at the end of the procedure.

• Additional procedure: When gallbladder stones are present, cholecystectomy is routinely performed at completion of the LSG procedure. The same trocars are used. Occasionally, in complicated cases, an additional 5-mm trocar is added 5-cm laterally to the right subcostal trocar.

6.2.4   Postoperative Management

Patients are mobilized on the same day of the operation and maintained with intravenous fluid therapy, proton pump inhibitors (PPIs), and analgesics. LMWH is administered subcutaneously 6 h after surgery and continued for 2 weeks. Short-term antibiotic therapy is added. Upper gastrointestinal contrast (Gastrografin) study is performed on the second postoperative day. Afterward, patients are put on a liquid diet and discharged on the fourth postoperative day. Soft diets with mashed and soft foods are prescribed for 4 weeks after surgery. One month after surgery, patients resume normal diet with the advice of adding one type of food at a time; meat may take longer to be tolerated. Five small meals a day are suggested. Postoperative follow-up is performed at 1, 3, 6, 12, 18, and 24 months after the operation and annually thereafter. Controls involve physical examination, blood tests (including vitamin B_1, B_{12}, folate, and serum iron, calcium, and vitamin D levels), upper gastrointestinal contrast (first month and first year), and liver ultrasound (sixth month). Endoscopic check is mandatory 2 years after the operation in all patients. Oral PPIs and ursodeoxycholic acid for 6 months, and multivitamin tablets for 1 year, are prescribed.

6.3   Results

6.3.1   Weight Loss

Short- to midterm outcomes of LSG in terms of weight loss are very good. According to the 2012 Fourth International Consensus Summit, accounting for 46,133 LSG performed by 130 surgeons worldwide, the percentage of excess weight loss (%EWL) at 1, 2, 3, 4, and 5 years was 59.3%, 59.0%, 54.7%, 52.3%, and 52.4%, respectively [21]. However, since LSG was approved as a stand-alone bariatric procedure only in 2009, long-term results from large series are lacking. In a recent review, Diamantis et al. reported on the 5-year results of nine studies enrolling 258 patients overall, with a mean %EWL of 62.3% [22].

Consistently, Sieber et al. showed a percentage of excess body mass index loss (%EBMIL) of 57.4% in their series of 54 patients 5 years after LSG [23]. These results seem to be maintained at a follow-up of ≥6 years; Eid et al. reported on a %EWL of 46% in 21 patients 8 years after LSG [14], while Sarela et al. showed a mean %EWL of 69% in 13 patients at a follow-up of 8 years or more [24].

We recently published the long-term results of our monocentric series of 148 patients with at least 6 years of follow-up; %EWL at 6 years was 67.3% and, a %EWL >50% (success rate) was achieved in 83.1% of patients. At a follow-up of ≥7 years, results were not significantly different (%EWL 65.7%; success rate 81%), confirming that the weight loss effect of this procedure is maintained over time [19].

6.3.2 Effect on Comorbidities

LSG is associated with a high rate of resolution of type 2 diabetes mellitus (T2DM) and other obesity-related comorbidities, such as arterial hypertension (AH) and obstructive sleep apnea (OSA) [25]. In the ASMBS 2009 position statement, accounting for 754 patients, T2DM remission ranged from 14 to 100%, AH from 15 to 93%, and OSA from 39 to 100% [7].

Weight loss and comorbidity resolution positively affect secondary cardiac structural and hemodynamic changes, referred to as obesity cardiomyopathy, including an increase in left-ventricular (LV) wall thickness, mass, and diameters, with systolic and diastolic dysfunction [26–29]. In our experience, LSG patients showed a significant change in LV shape in terms of mass, geometry, and diastolic function. These modifications were related to weight loss and to improvement of the metabolic syndrome, resulting in a significant reduction of the Framingham Risk Score [30].

Concerning T2DM, in several studies, 60–80% of diabetic obese patients undergoing LSG achieve remission of their pathology [31–34]. These results compared very favorably with those obtained after an intensive medical regimen [35] and were not statistically different from those after RYGB [36, 37]. The effectiveness of LSG on T2DM remission seems to be related to the functional reserve of β cells; in fact, diabetes postoperative duration >10 years, low C-peptide levels, and need for insulin therapy to control glycemia, are negative prognostic factors [38, 39]. In our series, T2DM remission occurred in 100% of patients with DM duration <10 years and in 31% with DM duration >10 years [38]. The beneficial action of LSG on T2DM occurs very early: Peterli et al. reported a significant modification of GLP-1 and PYY plasma levels 7 days after the procedure [40]. These results have been confirmed in a study by our group, which showed a significant increase of insulin secretion and sensitivity, plasma PYY, and GLP-1 just 72 h postoperatively, before the ingestion of any food [41]. At the same time, GHR values were significantly lower than those before the operation. Since GLP-1 and PYY are cosecreted from L cells in the small bowel in response of food ingestion, an intrinsic neurohormonal effect of LSG was suggested to explain these early changes. A gastric hypothesis was formulated [41], postulating that the diminished hydrochloric acid production induced by the significant reduction of oxyntic cell mass stimulates the vagally innervated antral mucosa, left intact by LSG, to secret gastrin-releasing peptide and, as a consequence, GLP-1 and PYY, without any food ingestion.

The long-term antidiabetic effects of LSG are not well documented due to the novelty of the procedure. In a small series of patients, at 5-year follow-up, remission was present in 87.8% of cases [42]. In our experience of 65 obese and diabetic patients submitted to LSG, remission was present in 57 patients (87%) and amelioration in 7 patients (10%) at a mean follow-up of 63 months (unpublished data). Most important, once remission was achieved, it was maintained in all cases except two, although weight regain occurred in six patients.

6.4 Complications (According to Clavien-Dindo Classification)

The postoperative mortality rate varies from 0.1 to 0.5% [21, 43, 44]. Early diagnosis is the most important factor to ensure a positive solution of complications, the management of which is often challenging and should be accomplished in bariatric centers by dedicated medical teams.

6.4.1 Bleeding (Grades II–IIIb)

Bleeding (1.1–8.7%) occurs most frequently within the first 24–48 h and almost always into the abdominal cavity, while it rarely determines hematemesis or melena [43, 45, 46]. More commonly, it originates from the staple line, in which case it increases the risk of gastric leak. Other sites of bleeding are the gastroepiploic and the short gastric vessels, which are divided during stomach mobilization, and trocar accesses. Hepatic or splenic injuries may cause severe postoperative bleeding if not recognized and managed intraoperatively. Once the hemodynamic parameters are stable, computed tomography (CT) scan is mandatory to define the bleeding site and quantify the hemoperitoneum. In case of hemorrhage from the staple line, CT images show a hematoma close to the gastric remnant. Bleeding can be self-limiting, requiring only blood transfusions, or it can be managed by interventional radiology. In case of massive uncontrolled hemorrhage, open or laparoscopic surgical exploration is mandatory. Suture line reinforcement has significantly reduced the occurrence of this complication [47].

6.4.2   Staple-Line Leak (Grades IIIa–IV)

Staple-line leak (0–7%) represents the most frequent complication after LSG, and it may be life-threatening. In most cases, leaks occur early, during the first postoperative week; late leaks (from the 8th to the ~40th postoperative day) are less frequent [13, 44].

Ninety percent of leaks occur just below the gastroesophageal junction (Fig. 6.4a). Both pathophysiological and technical factors seem to play a role in the development of gastric leaks after LSG. The former are represented by high intragastric pressure, sliding of the gastric tubule in the low-pressure mediastinum, lower thickness of the gastric fundus wall, and presence of a critical area of vascularization on the left side of the cardias region, where the oesophageal and gastric arterial systems are bordering [12]. Technical aspects include small bougie size (<36 F) and injury to the gastric wall during hemostasis or dissecting manoeuvers.

Practical rules are:

1. The staple line should not involve the critical area of vascularization, remaining 1–2 cm lateral to the angle of His (Fig. 6.3b).
2. The end of the staple line should be fixed to the left diaphragmatic pillar with two nonabsorbable sutures (Fig. 6.4b).
3. Countertraction should be somewhat loosened at the incisura angularis while resecting the stomach in order to avoid functional stenosis, which results in increased intragastric pressure (Fig. 6.4a).

The management of leaks is challenging, requiring a multidisciplinary approach, and it should be performed in experienced bariatric institutions. Timely diagnosis is the most important prognostic factor. Therefore, patients are advised to immediately contact the bariatric team in case of strange or unusual symptoms of any kind.

In our experience, operative treatment is reserved only for patients with hemodynamic instability and signs of acute peritonitis. Peritoneal toilet and proper drainage are recommended. Attempts to repair the fistula are contraindicated because of the high incidence of recurrence and the risk of adding further severe complications. In most cases, staple-line leaks can be successfully managed by percutaneous CT-guided drainage, alone or in combination with stent placement and enteral nutrition (Fig. 6.4c), without surgical intervention [48]. Unsuccessful control of the leak may require total gastrectomy or creation of a Roux limb.

Staple-line reinforcement seems to reduce the incidence of postoperative complications. To date, different reinforcement options have been proposed, such as oversewing the staple line with a running or inverting absorbable suture, buttressing the staple line with absorbable materials (bovine pericardium strips or porcine small intestine submucosa), and applying fibrin glue or hemostatic agents to the staple line. Routine reinforcement of the staple line, regardless of type, has been demonstrated to significantly reduce the incidence of bleeding. Data from a recent review, accounting for 8,920 patients, showed that buttressing

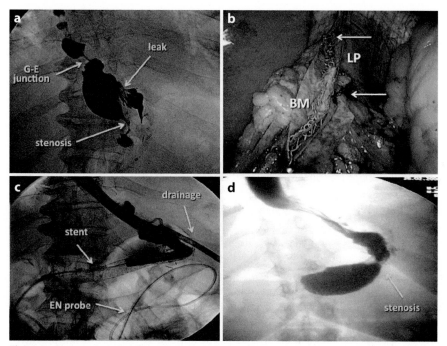

Fig. 6.4 a Upper gastric leak in patient with organic stenosis at the incisura angularis and dilation of the prestenosis segment. **b** Final end of the buttressing membrane is fixed to the left pillar by two nylon stitches (*arrows*). **c** Management of gastric leak using abdominal drainage, stent placement, and enteral nutrition. **d** Functional stenosis at the middle third of the gastric tubule. *LP* left pillar, *BM* buttressing membrane, *EN* enteral nutrition

the staple line with absorbable polymer membrane is more effective than other reinforcement methods for preventing gastric leaks [49].

6.4.3   Stenosis (Grades II–IIIb)

Stenosis (0.2–4%) usually it occurs at the transition between corpus and antrum of the gastric tubule, at the incisura angularis. It can be transient and related to transient dysmotility of the gastric muscular layers in this area, or it can be caused by incorrect orientation of the stapler during resection, resulting in an organic stenosis with long-lasting dysphagia and/or vomiting. A twisted sleeve may also cause symptomatic stenosis. An upper gastrointestinal contrast study is indicated to confirm gastric outlet obstruction (Fig. 6.4d). Endoscopy has both a diagnostic and therapeutic value. Repeated endoscopic dilations are the first approach, while placing endoscopic stents should be considered as an alternative solution.

In case of persistence of symptoms with nutrition problems, reoperation should be considered. Conversion to RYGB is the treatment of choice [50]. Laparoscopic seromyotomy of the stenotic tract (stricturoplasty) has also been proposed [51].

6.4.4 Gastroesophageal Reflux Disease (Grades II–IIIb)

The relationship between LSG and gastroesophageal reflux disease (GERD) is still a matter of discussion (varying from 0 to 30%). While in some published series postoperative improvement of GERD symptoms has been reported, in others, worsening has been noted [52–55]. The rationale of these conflicting data might be ascribed to the coexistence of different pathophysiological mechanisms, which could promote/worsen or improve GERD symptoms. The former entail lower esophageal sphincter (LES) malfunction due to section of sling fibers, sliding of the stomach tubule into the mediastinum determining diminished intraluminal pressure in the cardiac segment, increased intraluminal pressure in the gastric remnant, and delayed emptying of the stomach in case of mid-gastric stenosis of the lumen. The latter are represented by accelerated gastric emptying and reduced acid secretion. The presence of a hiatal hernia could also be associated with an increased risk of postoperative GERD development or worsening. Data concerning the effectiveness of hiatoplasty on GERD after LSG are not conclusive. However, in the Fourth International Consensus Summit on LSG held in 2012, there was general agreement that when a hiatal hernia is present, it should be repaired at the time of the bariatric procedure [21].

In a recent endoscopic survey of our patients submitted to LSG with a 3- to 5-year follow-up, a 15% incidence of peptic esophageal lesions and of nondysplastic Barrett's esophagus was found, with no correlation between the severity of reflux symptoms and the degree of esophageal lesions (unpublished data). These lesions were highly responsive to full-dose therapy with PPIs. For this reason, a careful postoperative follow-up schedule including an endoscopy within 2 years from the operation is recommended to our patients.

In patients complaining of reflux symptoms and not responsive to PPI therapy, conversion to RYGB is a valid option.

References

1. Hess DS, Hess DW (1998) Biliopancreatic diversion with a duodenal switch. Obes Surg 8:267–282
2. Scopinaro N, Gianetta E, Pandolfo N et al (1976) Bilio-pancreatic bypass. Proposal and preliminary experimental study of a new type of operation for the functional surgical treatment of obesity. Minerva Chir 31:560–566
3. Marceau P, Hould FS, Simard S et al (1998) Biliopancreatic diversion with duodenal switch. World J Surg 22:947–954

4. Ren CJ, Patterson E, Gagner M (2000) Early results of laparoscopic biliopancreatic diversion with duodenal switch: a case series of 40 consecutive patients. Obes Surg 10:514–523

5. Regan JP, Inabnet WB, Gagner M, Pomp A (2003) Early experience with two-stage laparoscopic Roux-en-Y gastric bypass as an alternative in the super-super obese patient. Obes Surg 13:861–864

6. Cottam D, Qureshi FG, Mattar SG et al (2006) Laparoscopic sleeve gastrectomy as an initial weight-loss procedure for high-risk patients with morbid obesity. Surg Endosc 20:859–863

7. Clinical Issues Committee of the American Society for Metabolic and Bariatric Surgery (2010) Updated position statement on sleeve gastrectomy as a bariatric procedure. Surg Obes Relat Dis 6:1–5

8. Karamanakos SN, Vagenas K, Kalfarentzos F, Alexandrides TK (2008) Weight loss, appetite suppression, and changes in fasting and postprandial ghrelin and peptide-YY levels after Roux-en-Y gastric bypass and sleeve gastrectomy: a prospective, double blind study. Ann Surg 247:401–407

9. Angrisani L, Santonicola A, Iovino P et al (2015) Bariatric surgery worldwide 2013. Obes Surg 25:1822–1832

10. Frezza EE, Chiriva-Internati M, Wachtel MS (2008) Analysis of the results of sleeve gastrectomy for morbid obesity and the role of ghrelin. Surg Today 38:481–483

11. Chabot F, Caron A, Laplante M, St-Pierre DH (2014) Interrelationships between ghrelin, insulin and glucose homeostasis: Physiological relevance. World J Diabetes 5:328–341

12. Basso N, Casella G, Rizzello M et al (2011) Laparoscopic sleeve gastrectomy as first stage or definitive intent in 300 consecutive cases. Surg Endosc 25:444–449

13. Rosenthal RJ; International Sleeve Gastrectomy Expert Panel, Diaz AA et al (2012) International Sleeve Gastrectomy Expert Panel Consensus Statement: best practice guidelines based on experience of >12,000 cases. Surg Obes Relat Dis 8:8–19

14. Eid GM, Brethauer S, Mattar SG et al (2012) Laparoscopic sleeve gastrectomy for super obese patients: forty-eight percent excess weight loss after 6 to 8 years with 93% follow-up. Ann Surg 256:262–265

15. Boza C, Daroch D, Barros D et al (2014) Long-term outcomes of laparoscopic sleeve gastrectomy as a primary bariatric procedure. Surg Obes Relat Dis 10:1129–1133

16. Weiner RA, Weiner S, Pomhoff I et al (2007) Laparoscopic sleeve gastrectomy – Influence of sleeve size and resected gastric volume. Obes Surg 17:1297–1305

17. Rawlins L, Rawlins MP, Brown CC, Schumacher DL (2013) Sleeve gastrectomy: 5-year outcomes of a single institution. Surg Obes Relat Dis 9:21–25

18. Atkins ER, Preen DB, Jarman C, Cohen LD (2012) Improved obesity reduction and co-morbidity resolution in patients treated with 40-French bougie versus 50-French bougie four years after laparoscopic sleeve gastrectomy. Analysis of 294 patients. Obes Surg 22:97–104

19. Casella G, Soricelli E, Giannotti D et al (2016) Long-term results after laparoscopic sleeve gastrectomy in a large monocentric series. Surg Obes Relat Dis 12:757–762

20. Casella G, Soricelli E, Fantini A, Basso N (2010) A time-saving technique for specimen extraction in sleeve gastrectomy. World J Surg 34:765–767

21. Gagner M, Deitel M, Erickson AL, Crosby RD (2013) Survey on laparoscopic sleeve gastrectomy (LSG) at the Fourth International Consensus Summit on Sleeve Gastrectomy. Obes Surg 23:2013–2017

22. Diamantis T, Apostolou KG, Alexandrou A et al (2014) Review of long-term weight loss results after laparoscopic sleeve gastrectomy. Surg Obes Relat Dis 10:177–183

23. Sieber P, Gass M, Kern B et al (2014) Five-year results of laparoscopic sleeve gastrectomy. Surg Obes Relat Dis 10:243–249

24. Sarela AI, Dexter SP, O'Kane M et al (2012) Long-term follow-up after laparoscopic sleeve gastrectomy: 8–9-year results. Surg Obes Relat Dis 8:679–684

25. Silecchia G, Boru C, Pecchia A et al (2006) Effectiveness of laparoscopic sleeve gastrectomy (first stage of biliopancreatic diversion with duodenal switch) on co-morbidities in super-obese high-risk patients. Obes Surg 16:1138–1144

26. Guh DP, Zhang W, Bansback N et al (2009) The incidence of co-morbidities related to obesity and overweight: a systematic review and meta-analysis. BMC Public Health 9:88

27. Sjöström L, Peltonen M, Jacobson P et al (2012) Bariatric surgery and long-term cardiovascular events. JAMA 307:56–65

28. Pascual M, Pascual DA, Soria F et al (2003) Effects of isolated obesity on systolic and diastolic left ventricular function. Heart 89:1152–1156

29. Wong CY, O'Moore-Sullivan T, Leano R et al (2004) Alterations of left ventricular myocardial characteristics associated with obesity. Circulation 110:3081–3087

30. Cavarretta E, Casella G, Calì B et al (2013) Cardiac remodeling in obese patients after laparoscopic sleeve gastrectomy. World J Surg 37:565–572

31. Abbatini F, Rizzello M, Casella G et al (2010) Long-term effects of laparoscopic sleeve gastrectomy, gastric bypass, and adjustable gastric banding on type 2 diabetes. Surg Endosc 24:1005–1010

32. Cottam D, Qureshi FG, Mattar SG et al (2006) Laparoscopic sleeve gastrectomy as an initial weight-loss procedure for high-risk patients with morbid obesity. Surg Endosc 20:859–863

33. Vidal J, Ibarzabal A, Romero F et al (2008) Type 2 diabetes mellitus and the metabolic syndrome following sleeve gastrectomy in severely obese subjects. Obes Surg 18:1077–1082

34. Cheverie J, Jacobsen GR, Sandler BJ et al (2013) Laparoscopic sleeve gastrectomy: an efficacious management of metabolic syndrome in the morbidly obese. Surg Endosc 27:S254

35. Leonetti F, Capoccia D, Coccia F et al (2012) Obesity, type 2 diabetes mellitus, and other comorbidities: a prospective cohort study of laparoscopic sleeve gastrectomy vs medical treatment. Arch Surg 147:694–700

36. Schauer PR, Burguera B, Ikramuddin S et al (2003) Effect of laparoscopic Roux-en Y gastric bypass on type 2 diabetes mellitus. Ann Surg 238:467–484

37. Buchwald H, Avidor Y, Braunwald E et al (2004) Bariatric surgery: a systematic review and meta-analysis. JAMA 292:1724–1737

38. Casella G, Abbatini F, Calì B et al (2011) Ten-year duration of type 2 diabetes as prognostic factor for remission after sleeve gastrectomy. Surg Obes Relat Dis 7:697–702

39. Lee WJ, Ser KH, Chong K et al (2010) Laparoscopic sleeve gastrectomy for diabetes treatment in nonmorbidly obese patients: efficacy and change of insulin secretion. Surgery 147:664–669

40. Peterli R, Wölnerhanssen B, Peters T et al (2009) Improvement in glucose metabolism after bariatric surgery: comparison of laparoscopic Roux-en-Y gastric bypass and laparoscopic sleeve gastrectomy: a prospective randomized trial. Ann Surg 250:234–241

41. Basso N, Capoccia D, Rizzello M et al (2011) First-phase insulin secretion, insulin sensitivity, ghrelin, GLP-1, and PYY changes 72 h after sleeve gastrectomy in obese diabetic patients: the gastric hypothesis. Surg Endosc 25:3540–3550

42. Abbatini F, Capoccia D, Casella G et al (2013) Long-term remission of type 2 diabetes in morbidly obese patients after sleeve gastrectomy. Surg Obes Relat Dis 9:498–502

43. Clinical Issues Committee of the American Society for Metabolic and Bariatric Surgery (2010) Updated position statement on sleeve gastrectomy as a bariatric procedure. Surg Obes Relat Dis 6:1–5

44. Deitel M, Gagner M, Erickson AL, Crosby RD (2011) Third International Summit: current status of sleeve gastrectomy. Surg Obes Relat Dis 7:749–759

45. Trastulli S, Desiderio J, Guarino S et al (2013) Laparoscopic sleeve gastrectomy compared with other bariatric surgical procedures: a systematic review of randomized trials. Surg Obes Relat Dis 9:816–829

46. Macias CA, Sandler B, Barajas-Gamboa JS et al (2013) Standardized protocol utilization decreases rate of complications: a study of laparoscopic sleeve gastrectomy in 189 consecutive patients. Surg Endosc 27:S489

47. D'Ugo S, Gentileschi P, Benavoli D et al (2014) Comparative use of different techniques for leak and bleeding prevention during laparoscopic sleeve gastrectomy: a multicenter study. Surg Obes Relat Dis 10:450–454

48. Casella G, Soricelli E, Rizzello M et al (2009) Nonsurgical treatment of staple line leaks after laparoscopic sleeve gastrectomy. Obes Surg 19:821–826

49. Gagner M, Buchwald JN (2014) Comparison of laparoscopic sleeve gastrectomy leak rates in four staple-line reinforcement options: a systematic review. Surg Obes Relat Dis 10:713–723

50. Parikh A, Alley JB, Peterson RM et al (2012) Management options for symptomatic stenosis after laparoscopic vertical sleeve gastrectomy in the morbidly obese. Surg Endosc 26:738–746

51. Vilallonga R, Himpens J, van de Vrande S (2013) Laparoscopic management of persistent strictures after laparoscopic sleeve gastrectomy. Obes Surg 23:1655–1661

52. Sheppard CE, Sadowski DC, de Gara CJ et al (2015) Rates of reflux before and after laparoscopic sleeve gastrectomy for severe obesity. Obes Surg 25:763–768

53. Rebecchi F, Allaix ME, Giaccone C et al (2014) Gastroesophageal reflux disease and laparoscopic sleeve gastrectomy: a physiopathologic evaluation. Ann Surg 260:909–915

54. Sharma A, Aggarwal S, Ahuja V, Bal C (2014) Evaluation of gastroesophageal reflux before and after sleeve gastrectomy using symptom scoring, scintigraphy, and endoscopy. Surg Obes Relat Dis 10:600–605

55. Laffin M, Chau J, Gill RS et al (2013) Sleeve gastrectomy and gastroesophageal reflux disease. J Obes 2013:741097

Roux-en-Y Gastric Bypass

7

Cristiano Giardiello, Pietro Maida, and Michele Lorenzo

7.1   Introduction

Bariatric surgery is actually considered the only therapeutic option in patients with morbid obesity who are affected by life-threatening comorbidities. Although a wide range of surgical bariatric options are offered, at this time, >50% of patients undergo a procedure based on the laparoscopic Roux-en-Y gastric bypass scheme [1].

In 1966, Mason and Ito first described the technique of laparotomic Roux-en-Y gastric bypass for treating morbid obesity [2]. In 1994, Wittgrove et al. reported the technique, and their preliminary experience with the laparoscopic Roux-en-Y gastric bypass (LRYGB) [3]. Since then, bariatric surgeons worldwide have made several modifications to the original technique in order to improve results and decrease complications. These technical changes were not accepted after randomized prospective studies but on the basis of the experience of individual bariatric surgeons and mutual collaboration with colleagues. Moreover, the biggest controversy regarding this procedure is the lack of clarity regarding its mechanism of action and its profound metabolic effect [4]. Variations in technical setup and operative procedures are without significant effects in term of safety and weight loss and mainly depend on surgeons' preferences (Table 7.1).

In this chapter, we describe two different technical approaches to LRYGB, both characterized by the absence of mesenteric section: the reverse technique and the double-loop technique.

C. Giardiello (✉)
General, Emergency and Metabolic Surgery Unit, Department of Surgery and Obesity Center, Pineta Grande Hospital
Castelvolturno, Italy
e-mail: cristiano.giardiello@pinetagrande.it

L. Angrisani (Ed), Bariatric and Metabolic Surgery,
Updates in Surgery
DOI: 10.1007/ 978-88-470-3944-5_7, © Springer-Verlag Italia 2017

Table 7.1 Laparoscopic Roux-en-Y gastric bypass: areas of surgical technical variation

Areas of surgical technical variation	
1. Alimentary limb position	a. Retrogastric or antegastric b. Retrocolic or antecolic
2. Length of alimentary and biliopancreatic limb	a. Alimentary limb – 100 cm – 150 cm –200 cm b. Biliopancreatic limb – 25 cm – 50 cm – 100 cm
3. Anastomosis technique	a. Hand sewn b. Circular stapler – endoesophageal assistance – endogastric assistance c. Linear stapler

7.2 Surgical Technique

7.2.1 Preoperative Patient Preparation

Appropriate preoperative surgical preparation is essential for the procedure. Intragastric balloon or liver shrinkage diet prior surgery is recommended, with the objective of reducing liver size and improving intraoperative visualization [5]. Prophylactic broad-spectrum intravenously administered antibiotics are routinely given at anesthesia induction and continued for several days, according to patient condition. Thromboprophylaxis is also done routinely using low-molecular-weight heparin preoperatively and then for 1–2 weeks postoperatively. Lower-limb pneumatic compression is also applied intraoperatively.

7.2.2 Patient and Surgeon Positioning

Patients are placed in the reverse Trendelenburg position with the split-leg approach. Usually, the operating surgeon stands between the patient's legs, with assistants on either side of the patient.

7.2.3 Pneumoperitoneum and Trocar Positioning

A 15- to 18-mmHg pneumoperitoneum is created by inserting a Veress needle into the left midclavicular line just below the costal margin. Five trocars are usually inserted: The first (T1) is inserted in the xiphoumbilical line 15 cm

Table 7.2 Laparoscopic surgical devices in each trocar

Trocar	Diameter	Reversal bypass	Double-loop bypass
T1	12 mm	Camera, graspers, ultrasonic devices	Camera
T2	12 mm	Camera, graspers, ultrasonic devices	Graspers, ultrasonic devices
T3	12 mm	Scissors, graspers	Scissors, graspers
T4	12 mm	Graspers, liver retractor, staplers	Liver retractor
T5	5–12 mm	Graspers, staplers	Graspers, staplers

below the sternum; usually, an optic trocar is used. The second (T2) is inserted in the left flank, in correspondence of crossing the umbilical transversal line with an anterior axillary line. The third (T3) is inserted in the front right upper quadrant a few centimeters below the costal margin in the midclavicular line. The fourth (T4) is positioned as T3 but in the right upper quadrant. The fifth (T5) is positioned a few centimeters under the xiphoid. Additional trocars can be positioned according to the patient's anatomy. Trocar diameter and laparoscopic devices used for each trocar are reported in Table 7.2.

7.2.4 Surgical Steps

7.2.4.1 Reverse Bypass

The first step is the creation of the jejunojejunal anastomosis. The biliopancreatic limb is prepared by jejunum sectioning with a linear stapler 1 m after the ligament of Treitz, avoiding the mesentery opening. The alimentary limb is measured at 1.5 m from the section and a laterolateral jejunojejunostomy is performed by firing a 45-cm blue cartridge. The enterotomies are closed using a 2/0 absorbable monofilament running suture. The following step is creating the gastric pouch. The liver is retracted and blunt/ultrasonic dissection is started at the angle of His. A window is created between the first and second vessel of the lesser curve 6 cm from the cardias. A horizontal section of the stomach is created using a blue cartridge. A vertical stapler is inserted to create the pouch. The gastrojejunal anastomosis is performed by a single firing of a 45-cm linear blue cartridge. Methylene blue test is done to check for leaks (Figs. 7.1–7.3).

7.2.4.2 Double-Loop Technique

First, the 30-cc tube is inserted into the esophagus for evacuating any intragastric air or small residual gastric content and is retracted at the cardias level to guide the surgical maneuver. All these maneuvers are blunt or with ultrasonic dissection. The angle of His is prepared posteriorly just lateral to the left diaphragmatic crus and anteriorly as deep as possible. Blunt and ultrasonic dissection is done on the lesser sac to access the epiploon retrocavity (4–5 cm below the gastroesophageal junction). After freeing all adhesions, a linear articulated stapler is inserted perpendicularly to the lesser curvature to cut the stomach horizontally. Usually,

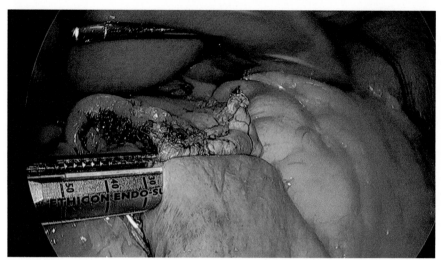

Fig. 7.1 Reverse Roux-en-Y gastric bypass. Gastrojejunal anastomosis with linear stapler

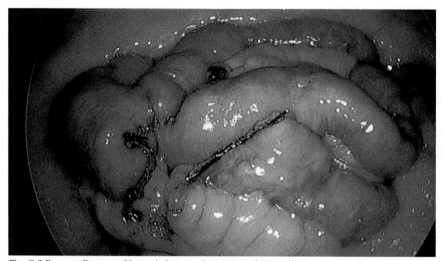

Fig. 7.2 Reverse Roux-en-Y gastric bypass. Laterolateral jejunoileal anastomosis

and depending on gastric thickness, a 60-mm blue cartridge is used. The pouch is created by vertically firing a 60-mm cartridge inserted toward the angle of His, along the gastric tube, starting from the most lateral point of the horizontal transection line.

The gastrojejunostomy is created starting at the individuation of Treitz while looking for a loop mobile enough to reach the anastomotic site without abnormal tension. A gastrojejunal laterolateral antecolic procedure with linear stapler (60

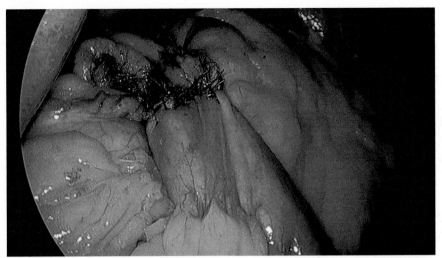

Fig. 7.3 Reverse Roux-en-Y gastric bypass. Stapler accesses closed at the end of gastrojejunal anastomosis

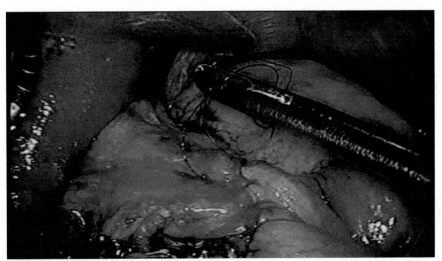

Fig. 7.4 Double-loop Roux-en-Y gastric bypass. Gastrojejunal anastomosis with closure of stapler accesses

mm) is then performed (first loop). Enterotomic access for the stapler is closed with an absorbable running suture.

The ileojejunal anastomosis starts with measuring a 150- to 200-cm alimentary limb. A laterolateral ileojejunal (second loop) anastomosis is performed with a 60-mm white cartridge. Enterotomies are closed, the last white cartridge is fired between the two anastomosis to divide the jejunal loop and create the Roux-en-Y, and the methylene blue test is performed at the end of the procedure (Figs. 7.4–7.6).

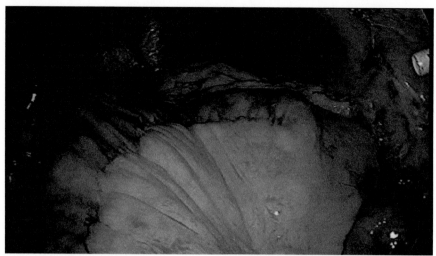

Fig. 7.5 Double-loop Roux-en-Y gastric bypass. On the left the jejunal loop still unsectioned, on the right the gastrojejunal anastomosis

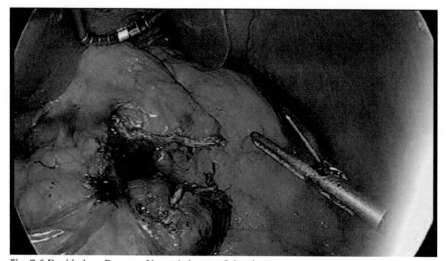

Fig. 7.6 Double-loop Roux-en-Y gastric bypass. Jejunal stumps

7.3   **Complications** (According to Clavien-Dindo Classification)

After LRYGB, several significant and potentially catastrophic complication can occur (Table 7.3). The overall complication rate, reported in a recent systematic review with meta-analysis, is ~21% (12–33%) [6]. The reoperation rate is 3–20% and mortality rate ~0.38% (<30 days) and 0.72% (>30 days). Early complications

Table 7.3 Laparoscopic Roux-en-Y gastric bypass: incidence and timing of main complication presentation

Complication	Rate (%)	Timing [a]
Bleeding	0.8–4.4	Early
Leak	1–2	Early/Intermediate
Obstruction [b]	1–5	Late
Ulcers	4	Late
Strictures	5	Late

[a] Early, <1 week; intermediate, 1 week–1 month; late, >1 month
[b] Regarding reversal bypass and double-loop bypass; in the authors' experience, this complication is absent

tend to be related to technical issue; late complications tend to include metabolic or nutritional problems. Clavien-Dindo classification is inserted to compare outcome data among different centers [7].

7.3.1 Gastrointestinal Bleeding (Grade IIa)

The rate of gastrointestinal bleeding after gastric bypass is 0.8–4.4%. This complication can start from anywhere in the gastrointestinal tract, and it may be clinically expressed by hematemesis, melena, or intraperitoneal bleeding. These manifestations are usually accompanied by early tachycardia and tachypnea, abdominal pain, or distension. The gastrojejunal anastomosis is considered the most frequently involved site after LRYGB. A conservative treatment with intravenously applied liquid infusion and blood transfusion is usually therapeutic following minimal blood loss. In massive hemorrhages, a laparoscopic or laparotomic attempt is mandatory [6, 8–10].

7.3.2 Leak (Grade III)

Anastomotic and staple-line leak can result in high morbidity rates. Fistulas, peritonitis, abscess formation, sepsis, and multiorgan failure can be all observed as life-threatening consequences after a leak. Leak occurs more frequently in gastrojejunal anastomosis and occurs less frequently in the staple-line margin.

Intraoperative diagnosis is usually performed using the methylene blue test. Postoperatively, a leak must be suspected by the clinical presence of tachycardia (>120 bpm), tachypnea, fever, abdominal pain, hypotension, and hiccup. Upper gastrointestinal contrast studies with gastrografin are usually able to precisely reveal the presence and site of a leak. Therapeutic approach can be conservative, with a nasogastric tube, fluids, and antibiotics; and endoscopic stent is the most frequently performed therapeutic option, and only in unsuccessful cases is laparoscopic closure of the defect indicated. Only in rare cases with unsuccessful conservative, endoscopic, and laparoscopic attempts a total gastrectomy is mandatory. Staple line reinforcement is proven to be effective for preventing this complication [6, 11–13].

7.3.3   Bowel Occlusion (Grade IIIb)

Intestinal occlusion in bariatric surgery is considered a complication specifically related to the LRYGB. The rate of this complication is 1.5–5%, and most cases were diagnosed during the first 12 months after surgery. Then, the incidence slowly decreased until 42–48 months postoperatively. This complication, in particular, occurs more frequently in the laparoscopic than in the laparotomic approach. This fact is probably linked to the absence of mesenteric opening without scares. The bowel can move freely into the abdomen without provoking obstruction or entering new open mesenteric spaces (Petersen space). In the double-loop or reverse bypass technique, the mesenterium is not open, and this complication is never observed. The clinical presentation of bowel obstruction in patients who underwent LRYGB is different than in nonobese patients. Due to the small volume of the gastric pouch, vomit volume is scarce, while vague abdominal discomfort or colic are more frequently observed. The diagnosis is usually made by CT scan with gastrografin, and the only therapy is surgical [6, 14, 15].

7.3.4   Stricture (Grades IIIa, IIIb)

The anastomotic stricture rate after LRYGB is 5% and occurs primarily at the site of the gastrojejunal anastomosis. This complication is usually related to marginal ulcer scar and tension and ischemia on anastomotic stumps. The 21-mm circular stapler is now considered in the pathogenesis of this complication. Usually, the clinical presentation of anastomotic stricture is characterized by nausea, vomiting, and dysphagia one or more months after surgery. The gold standard of gastrojejunal anastomosis treatment is endoscopic dilatation. Only in unsuccessful cases is it necessary to perform a laparoscopic revision. Rarely a stricture is localized near the jejunojejunal anastomosis. Clinical presentation is not substantially different, and a laparoscopic revision must be performed [6, 16].

7.4   Results

LRYGB results in significant early weight loss, which is partially maintained after longer follow-up. Most data come from a meta-analysis of Buchwald et al., which reports 62% excess weight loss (%EWL) and 0.5% 30-day mortality rate [17].

Most patients are expected to lose >50% of their excess weight. Weight loss is maximal at 2 years (32%) and declines during the following years (25%). Compared with conservative treatment, the Swedish Obesity Study (SOS) demonstrated better results in operated patients than in patients with dietetic treatment or who underwent vertical banded gastroplasty or laparoscopic adjustable gastric banding [18]. These results were confirmed in randomized controlled trials, as described by Angrisani et al., who compared LRYGB and laparoscopic adjustable gastric banding (LAGB) [19]. Long-term comparative results with laparoscopic sleeve gastrectomy (LSG) are lacking. Technically different approaches to gastric bypass do not seem to be considerably different in terms of weight loss and comorbidities, as observed for mini-gastric bypass, reverse bypass, and the double-loop technique.

Improvement in obesity-related comorbidities is considered strictly proportional to weight loss [17], and some observations regarding improvement in comorbidities have recently been related to the type of bariatric procedure [17, 20, 21]. This is the case with type 2 diabetes mellitus and gastroesophageal reflux disease. In these conditions, a specific role for RYGB was discovered, which is probably linked to the new anatomy of the digestive tract after surgery. Gastric bypass appears to have superior effects on type 2 diabetes remission to other restrictive procedures, such as LAGB or LSG. These effects are mainly related to duodenal exclusion, or switch. Buchwald et al., in a meta-analysis study, showed that diabetes improved in 80%, 57%, and 95% of patients treated with gastric bypass, gastric banding, or duodenal switch, respectively [17]. Lee et al., in a randomized controlled trial, studied the effects of RYGB and LSG in patients with a body mass index (BMI) of 25–35 kg/m^2 [22]. They observed that diabetic patients who underwent RYGB achieved greater disease remission than LSG patients (93 vs. 43%). More recently, the STAMPEDE (Surgical Treatment and Medications Potentially Eradicate Diabetes Efficiently) trial reported 3-year follow-up results comparing poorly controlled diabetic patients who underwent RYGB, LSG, or medical treatment [23]. Glycated hemoglobin (HbA1c) <6.0% was observed in 51% of patients who underwent RYGB, 37% of those treated with LSG, and 24.5% of those treated medically. The Diabetes Surgery Randomized Controlled Trial demonstrated that, in patients with BMI 30–39.9 kg/m^2, RYGB resulted in HBA1c <7%, low-density lipoprotein cholesterol <100 mg/dL, systolic blood pressure <130 mmHg in 49%, while similar results were achieved in only 19% of patients under medical treatment [24]. Adams et al., in two different trials, demonstrated a significant improvement in major cardiovascular and metabolic risk factors after RYGB compared with more invasive procedures [25, 26].

Nonalcoholic fatty liver disease (NAFLD) is common in morbidly obese patients. In the majority of patients with this disease who underwent RYGB resulted in a reduction of steatosis grade, liver inflammation, and fibrosis [27]. Moreover, the real role of bariatric surgery in patients with this disease is still a matter of concern, and NAFLD alone in not currently considered an indication for RYGB.

Is still unclear whether the high remission rate (66%) of sleep apnea and other respiratory disorders obtained in patients who underwent RYGB is strictly linked to weight loss or whether there is an added effect from the procedure.

7.5   Conclusions

LRYGB provides an excellent and prolonged excess weight loss and resolution or improvement of life-threatening comorbidities, such as diabetes. It is the procedure of choice for patients with preexisting gastroesophageal efflux disease and is considered safe, with a low risk of anastomotic bleeding and other complications. Several variations of surgical technique have been suggested over the years according to surgeon experience and preferences. The laparoscopic reversal bypass and the double-loop laparoscopic bypass have similar efficacy and a very low risk of intestinal hernia and occlusion.

References

1.   Angrisani L, Lorenzo M (2014) Bariatric surgery worldwide: overview and results. In: Foletto M, Rosenthal RJ (eds) The Globesity challenge to general surgery. Springer, Milan, pp 237–246
2.   Mason EE, Ito C (1967) Gastric bypass in obesity. Surg Clin North Am 47:1345–1351
3.   Wittgrove AC, Clark GW, Tremblay LJ (1994) Laparoscopic gastric bypass. Roux-en-Y: preliminary report of five cases. Obes Surg 4:435–437
4.   Pedersen SD (2013) The role of hormonal factors in weight loss and recidivism after bariatric surgery. Gastroenterol Res Pract 52:428–450
5.   Genco A, Bruni T, Doldi SB et al (2005) BioEnterics intragastric balloon: the Italian experience with 2,515 patients. Obes Surg 15:1161–1164
6.   Chang SH, Stoll CR, Song J et al (2014) The effectiveness and risks of bariatric surgery: an updated systematic review and meta-analysis, 2003–2012. JAMA Surg 149:275–287
7.   Dindo D, Demartines N, Clavien PA (2004) Classification of surgical complications. A new proposal with evaluation in a cohort of 6336 patients and results of survey. Ann Surg 240:205–213
8.   Thomas H, Agraval S (2012) Systematic review of obesity surgery mortality risk score – preoperative risk stratification in bariatric surgery. Obes Surg 22:1135–1140
9.   Mehran A, Szomstein S, Zundel N, Rosenthal R (2003) Management of acute bleeding after laparoscopic Roux-en-Y gastric bypass. Obes Surg 13:842–847
10.   Angrisani L, Lorenzo M, Borrelli V et al (2004) The use of bovine pericardial strips on linear stapler to reduce extraluminal bleeding during laparoscopic gastric bypass: prospective randomized clinical trial. Obes Surg 14:1198–1202
11.   Chousleb E, Szomstein S, Podkameni D et al (2004) Routine abdominal drains after laparoscopic Roux-en-Y gastric bypass: a retrospective review of 593 patients. Obes Surg 14:1203–1207
12.   Dillemans B, Skran N, Van Cauvenberge S et al (2009) Standardization of the fully stapled laparoscopic Roux-en-Y gastric bypass for obesity reduces early immediate postoperative morbidity and mortality: a single-center study on 2606 patients. Obes Surg 19:1355–1364

13. Brockmeyer JR, Simon TE, Jakob RK et al (2012) Upper gastrointestinal swallow study following bariatric surgery: institutional review and review of the literature. Obes Surg 22:1039–1043

14. Hussin S, Ahmed AR, Johnson J et al (2007) Small-bowel obstruction after laparoscopic Roux-en-Y gastric bypass: etiology, diagnosis, and management. Arch Surg 142:988–993

15. Higa KD, Ho T, Boone KB (2003) Internal hernias after laparoscopic Roux-en-Y gastric bypass: incidence treatment and prevention. Obes Surg 13: 350–354

16. Ukleja A, Afonso BB, Pimentel R et al (2008) Outcome of endoscopic balloon dilatation of strictures after laparoscopic gastric bypass. Surg Endosc 22:1746–1750

17. Buchwald H, Avidor Y, Braunwals E et al (2004) Bariatric surgery: a systematic review and meta-analysis. JAMA 292:1724–1732

18. Sjostrom L (2013) Review of the key results from the Swedish Obese Subjects (SOS) trial – A prospective controlled intervention study of bariatric surgery. J Intern Med 273:219–234

19. Angrisani L, Lorenzo M, Borrelli V (2007) Laparoscopic adjustable gastric banding versus Roux-en-Y gastric bypass: 5-year results of a prospective randomized trial. Surg Obes Relat Dis 3:127–132

20. Li JF, Lai DD, Lin ZH et al (2014) Comparison of the long-term results of Roux-en-Y gastric bypass and sleeve gastrectomy for morbid obesity: a systematic review and meta-analysis of randomized and nonrandomized trials. Surg Laparosc Endosc Percutan Tech 24:1–11

21. Angrisani L, Iovino P, Lorenzo M et al (1999) Treatment of morbid obesity and gastroesophageal reflux with hiatal hernia by LAP-BAND. Obes Surg 9:396–398

22. Lee WJ, Chong K, Ser KH et al (2011) Gastric bypass vs sleeve gastrectomy for type 2 diabetes mellitus: a randomized controlled trial. Arch Surg 146:143–148

23. Schauer PR, Bhatt DL, Kirwan JP et al (2014) Bariatric surgery versus intensive medical therapy for diabetes: 3 years outcomes. N Engl J Med 370:2002–2013

24. Ikramuddin S, Korner J, Lee WI et al (2012) Roux-en-Y gastric bypass vs intensive medical management for the control of type 2 diabetes, hypertension, and hyperlipidemia: The Diabetes Surgery Study Randomized Trial. JAMA 309:2240–2249

25. Adams TD, Davidson LE, Litwin SE et al (2012) Health benefit of gastric bypass surgery after 6 years. JAMA 308:1122–1131

26. Adams TD, Gress RE, Smith SS et al (2007) Long-term mortality after gastric bypass surgery. N Engl J Med 357:753–761

27. Hafeez S, Ahmed NH (2013) Bariatric surgery as potential treatment for non-alcoholic fatty liver disease: a future treatment by choice or by chance? J Obes 2013:839275

Mini-Gastric Bypass/One Anastomosis Gastric Bypass

8

Maurizio De Luca, Emilio Manno, Mario Musella, and Luigi Piazza

8.1   Introduction

The concept of a gastric bypass, consisting of one anastomosis, was first introduced by Mason in 1967 [1]. In this early configuration, the gastric pouch was very high, short, and had a horizontal shape, exposing the esophageal mucosa to caustic alkaline bile reflux coming from the jejunal loop (Fig. 8.1). It was therefore abandoned soon. Nevertheless, the spread of laparoscopic surgery led Rutledge to return to this concept by introducing in 1997 a different version of a single anastomosis gastric bypass, which he named the mini-gastric bypass (MGB). It consisted of a laterolateral anastomosis between a long-sleeved gastric pouch starting at the level of the crow's foot and a jejunal loop approximately 180–250 cm distal from the duodenal ligament of Treitz [2] (Fig. 8.2). A technical variation was then proposed in 2005 by a Spanish group with the definition of one anastomosis gastric bypass (OAGB) [3]. Since then, other names, such as single anastomosis gastric bypass (SAGB) or omega loop gastric bypass (OLGB) have been proposed to define this same technique [4, 5]. This confusion led a group of surgeons especially experienced with this technique to suggest in 2013 the name mini-gastric bypass/one anastomosis gastric bypass (MGB/OAGB) to define this surgery [6].

When presented in 2001, MGB/OAGB raised several doubts due to the predictable high rate of two worrisome complications: bile reflux in the short term, and gastric-pouch cancer over the long term [7]. These were attributed to the proposed technique, which comprised a single-loop anastomosis, thus resembling the Billroth II reconstruction following subtotal gastrectomy. However, it must be remarked that although some bariatric surgeons still confound the two techniques, MGB/OAGB from a technical point of view is

M. De Luca (✉)
Department of Surgery, Montebelluna Treviso Hospital
Montebelluna, Italy
e-mail: nnwdel@tin.it

L. Angrisani (Ed), Bariatric and Metabolic Surgery,
Updates in Surgery
DOI: 10.1007/ 978-88-470-3944-5_8, © Springer-Verlag Italia 2017

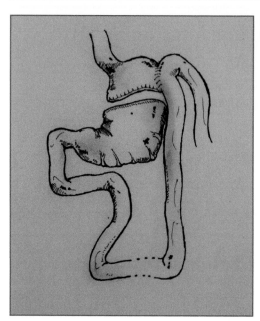

Fig. 8.1 The original Mason's loop bypass

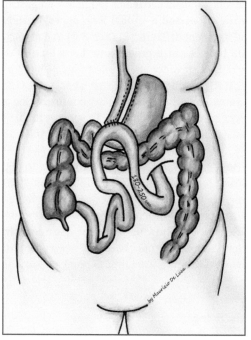

Fig. 8.2 The mini-gastric bypass/one anastomosis gastric bypass (MGB/OAGB)

definitely not the old loop gastric bypass proposed by Mason in 1967 [1]. The differences between the two techniques are well depicted in Figs. 8.1 and 8.2. Furthermore, high rates of bile reflux, often expected by opponents, have been rarely reported by MGB/OAGB performers and does not exceed 2% of all operated patients [4, 7]. Conversely, an interesting systematic review showed the risk of esophagogastric cancer to be extremely low following bariatric surgery and to be unknown following MGB/OAGB [8].

MGB/OAGB appears extremely effective in reducing obesity-related comorbidities, offering a good quality of life with a very acceptable complication rate [9]. Although not officially recognized in the USA as a bariatric procedure, the trend in the use of MGB/OAGB in Europe and Asia Pacific is rapidly growing [10], placing it as the most frequently performed procedure following sleeve gastrectomy (SG), Roux-en-Y gastric bypass (RYGB), and adjustable gastric banding (AGB).

8.2 Technique

MGB/OAGB is routinely performed with a standard five-port laparoscopic technique. Patients are placed in the reverse Trendelenburg position with legs spread. At the beginning of the operation, the surgeon stands between the patient's legs in order to prepare the phrenogastric ligament then, in some cases, moves to the right side of the patient. The monitor is at the head of the operating table and in some cases on the left side of the patient. The operation consists of two steps: a long-sleeved gastric tube along the lesser curvature and a Billroth type II loop gastrojejunostomy with a 180- to 250-cm afferent limb.

8.2.1 Long and Narrow Gastric Pouch

The first trocar – for the camera – is placed in the midpoint between the xiphoid and the umbilicus. The second trocar is placed in the right hypochondrium, the third is inserted in the left hypochondrium, symmetrical to the previous one, the fourth just under the xiphoid process, and the fifth in the right quadrant at mid-clavicular line on the same level of the camera [11]. A long gastric tube is the cornerstone of this procedure, placing the single anastomosis of a loop bypass away from the esophagocardial junction and thereby avoiding the problem of bile esophagitis that occurs with the original Mason's loop gastric bypass [1]. The gastric tube should be constructed as long and narrow as possible and is usually created by applying one horizontal 45-mm roticulator linear stapler at the angle of the lesser curvature, just above the left branch of the crow's foot. Multiple vertical 60-mm roticulator linear staple cartridges are placed upward to the angle of His and calibrated along a 32- to 36-Fr bougie, similar to the vertical part of a SG [5]. A 28- to 36-Fr bougie is strongly recommended for controlling the width of the tube. A narrow tube may help avoid weight regain and may also reduce acid production and so decrease the risk of marginal ulcer [4]. Although some data indicate that a running absorbable seromuscular-seromuscular invagination suture protects against leakage [3], no reinforcement was routinely done on the staple line.

8.2.2   Gastrojejunostomy

At this point, the surgeon begins the second part of the procedure, moving the omentum upward. Sectioning of the greater omentum into a bivalve is rarely needed. The jejunum is then identified at the ligament of Treitz and measured with a graded grasper to 180–250 cm from the Treitz ligament according to the patient's preoperative body mass index (BMI), previous operations, and alimentary behavior. The proximal limb should be always placed on the patient's left side and distal limb on the right to avoid torsion of the intestinal mesentery [4]. The original Rutledge technique is an end-to-side anastomosis, but most surgeons prefer a side-to-side technique, with the afferent limb higher than the efferent loop so as to form an isoperistalsis conduit [2, 4, 5]. Some surgeons have proposed placing an anchoring suture for the afferent limb on the staple line of the gastric pouch, with 6 to 10 sutures acting as a valve to inhibit bile reflux [3, 7]. An antecolic terminolateral gastrojejunostomy is performed using a posterior 45-mm Roticulator linear stapler and an anterior running suture or a continuous manual suture with an adsorbable suture. The anastomosis is created with a size of 1.5–3 cm, which is wider than for the RYGB because the restriction is provided by the narrow-sleeved tube rather than the small anastomosis used in RYGB [4]. Anastomosis is checked by intraoperative methylene blue test. Some authors introduce a nasogastric tube into the efferent loop, and some place a drain close to the anastomosis until the second postoperative day.

8.3   Results

8.3.1   Weight Loss and Weight-Related Disease

Rutledge reported a percentage of excess weight loss (%EWL) of 77% at 24 months in a series of 1274 cases [2]. Carbajo et al. reported a %EWL of 80% at 24 months considering a series of 209 patients [3]. Noun et al. considered 1000 patients who underwent OAGB with a mean of 5-year follow-up; %EWL was 72.5%. The 50%EWL was achieved for 95% of patients at 18 months and for 89.8% at 60 months. Operative time was 89 min, and length of hospital stay was 1.85 days for primary surgery and 2.35 for revision surgery [11]. Bruzzi et al. reported a 5-year postoperative percentage of excess body mass index loss (%EBMIL) of 71.5 ± 26.5% in 175 patients who underwent to OAGB. Postoperative gastrointestinal quality of life index (GIQLI) score of the treatment group was significantly higher than the preoperative score of the control group (110.3 ± 17.4 vs. 92.5 ± 15.9; $p<0.001$) [9]. Musella and the Italian Multicenter Study Group reported a %EWL of 77% considering 974 OAGB patients and a 5-year follow-up rate of 83.9% [7].

Lee et al. compared weight loss following RYGB patients with 40.5% preoperative BMI and OAGB patients with 41.1% preoperative BMI. At the fifth postoperative year, the %EWL was 58.7% for the RYGB group and 64.9% for the OAGB group. The residual excess weight <50% at 2 years was achieved in 75% of the RYGB group and 95% of the OAGB group. Operative morbidity was higher in RYGB group (20% vs. 7.5%). The authors evaluated hospital stay, which was longer in RYGB group (6.9 vs. 5.5 day) and cumulative dose of analgesic medication, which was larger in the RYGB group (3.4 vs. 2.0 doses). A significant improvement in obesity-related clinical parameters and complete resolution of metabolic syndrome in both groups were noted. GIQLI increased significantly without any significant difference between groups [12]. The same authors then evaluated two groups of patients – RYGB and OAGB – after 10 years of experience and with a follow-up of 1–10 years. Major complications were higher for the RYGB group (3.2% vs. 1.8%). At 5 years postoperatively, RYGB and OAGB patients had a BMI of 27.7 and 29.2, kg/m² respectively; %EWL was 60.1% vs. 72.9%. There were no significant differences in GIQLI score at 5 years between groups [13]. Quan et al. conducted a comprehensive literature search by retrieving the databases of PubMed, EMBASE, and the Cochrane Library and identified 16 studies for systematic review and 15 articles for meta-analysis. They compared OAGB with laparoscopic adjustable gastric banding (LAGB), laparoscopic SG (LSG), and laparoscopic RYGB (LRYGB). OAGB showed significantly higher weight loss compared to LAGB, LSG, and LRYGB [14].

8.3.2   Type 2 Diabetes Mellitus and Comorbidities

Lee et al., in a retrospective study of 443 patients with a BMI >35 kg/m² and 12-month follow-up (100% of patients) evaluated fasting plasma glucose (FPG) and glycated hemoglobin (HbA1c). FPG reached normal range in 89.5% of patients and HbA1c lowered to <7% in 76.5% of patients; 90% of type 2 diabetes mellitus (T2DM) patients came off their medication, and there was a significant improvement in lipid levels [15]. In a retrospective study of 62 patients with a very low BMI (23–35 kg/m²) and 24-month follow-up (100% of patients), the same authors recorded that BMI ranged from 30.1 to 23 kg/m², FPG from 195 to 106 mg/dL, and HbA1c from 9.7% to 5.9%; 55% of patients were off their T2DM medication at the final follow-up [16]. In the meta-analysis and systematic review by Quan et al., OAGB showed comparable or better results regarding T2DM remission versus LAGB, LSG, and LRYGB [14].The Italian Multicenter Study

Group reported T2DM remission of 84.4% and hypertension resolution of 87.5% in 974 OAGB patients at 60-month follow-up [7]. Finally, a recent multicenter European study [17] has shown the efficacy of both MGB/OAGB and LSG in determining T2DM remission at 12 months. This paper suggested that T2DM remission is independent from weight loss, with MGB/OAGB outperforming LSG on univariate analysis.

8.4 Complications (According to Clavien-Dindo Classification)

8.4.1 Early complications

8.4.1.1 Gastrointestinal bleeding (Grades IIIa, IIIb)
Gastrointestinal anastomosis bleeding should be suspected in the presence of hemodynamic instability and decrease of hemoglobin levels if no signs of abdominal bleedings are present. Most cases are treated by endoscopy with adrenaline injection, clips, and stitches at the bleeding source. Chevallier et al. reported only one case of gastrointestinal bleeding from the anastomosis in >1000 patients treated endoscopically [5].

8.4.1.2 Leak (Grade IIIb)
Gastrointestinal leak is probably the most fearsome complication in MGB/OAGB. Due to the presence of a high flux of bile coming from the afferent loop, anastomosis leak often causes a clinical onset of choleperitoneum that requires immediate surgical revision. Surgical strategy depends on the extent of the defect. In the presence of a large defect, conversion to RYGB could be the best choice. If the defect is small, primary closure can give good results. In addition to gastrointestinal anastomosis, leakage coming from the gastric pouch and gastric remnant have been described [7], with an incidence ranging from 0.6 to 1.8% [18].

8.4.1.3 Abdominal Bleeding (Grades II–IIIb)
The most frequent cause of abdominal bleeding is bleeding from trocar insertion sites. Frequency ranges from 0.1 to 2.5% [5]. Bleeding following spleen injury is very rare.

8.4.1.4 Peritonitis (Grade IIIb)
Peritonitis is caused by small-bowel mobilization using the grasper during the laparoscopic procedure and always requires surgical revision. The strategy is related to the distance from the gastrointestinal anastomosis. Conversion to RYGB is indicated if the perforation is close to the gastrointestinal junction [5]. Primary closure and drainage is recommended in all the other cases.

8.4.2 Late Complications

8.4.2.1 Bile Reflux (Grades II–IIIb)

Bile reflux is the most notoriously controversial disadvantage of MGB/OAGB. Prejudice arose from Mason's loop gastric bypass, after which bilious vomiting and subsequent gastritis and esophagitis were reported in 70% of patients. This may occur in the old Mason's gastric bypass with a small, high gastric pouch and alkaline reflux esophagitis due to a loop adjacent to the esophagus [1] (Fig. 8.1). However, there is a great difference between the Mason's procedure and MGB, with anastomosis in the latter being made on a long, narrow gastric pouch far from the esophagus. Chevallier et al. evaluated bile reflux by endoscopic biopsies in MGB/OAGB patients. The authors registered, as a sign of bile reflux, foveolar dysplasia only in 17.1% of patients at 2 years and 4.6% at 4 years, with no dysplasia or metaplasia. Bile reflux, if present, is not symptomatic in all patients [5]. Symptoms (heartburn, dyspepsia, bilious vomiting) can be successfully treated pharmacologically in most cases. Bile reflux rarely needs surgical revision. If revision is needed, conversion to RYGB is the treatment of choice.

8.4.2.2 Anastomotic Ulcer (Grades II–IIIb)

Anastomotic ulcers are often caused by the small gastric pouch continuing to secrete acids. Heavy cigarette smoking and and stopping proton pump inhibitor (PPI) therapy might play a role. A larger gastric pouch with more acid secretions could be related to the incidence of ulcers. Treatment strategy is related to clinical onset, and continuing PPI therapy and quitting smoking in cases with clinical and endoscopic findings are recommended. Although rare, an untreated anastomotic ulcer can perforate, causing clinic onset of peritonitis. In these case, conservative treatment with a T tube [5] or a new gastrojejunal anastomosis and RYGB conversion are treatments of choice [14].

8.4.2.3 Iron Deficiency (Grade II)

MGB often causes microcytic anemia. This because in MGB/OAGB, a longer bypass is created in the foregut limb compared with in RYGB, which more severely inhibits iron absorption. In all cases, iron therapy i.v. is the treatment of choice.

8.4.2.4 Protein Malnutrition (Grades II–IIIb)

A well-recognized late complication is protein malnutrition. Clinical signs are albuminemia <30 g/L, %EBMIL >100%, and BMI <20 kg/m². The first treatment is conservative. If ineffective, surgical MGB/OAGB reversal is the treatment of choice [5]. Lee et al. [18] suggests conversion of MGB/OAGB to SG, with good effect on malnutrition and no weight regain.

8.4.2.5 Internal Hernia (Grade IIIb)

A worrisome complication – internal hernia – often presents with insidious and non-specific symptoms that may be difficult to assess clinically. Single anastomosis of MGB/OAGB reduces potential sites of internal hernias. Although the incidence of this complication after MGB/OAGB is very rare, some experts suggest closing the Petersen space as well.

8.4.2.6 Weight Regain (Grade IIIb)

If weight regain is associated with gastric pouch dilatation, revision surgery by pouch trimming on a calibration tube is indicated. Other techniques are RYGB conversion with a 150-cm alimentary limb or efferent loop shortening to increase the malabsorptive component of MGB. Incidence ranges from 0.8 to 5% [18].

8.4.2.7 Cancer (Grade IIIb)

In the mid-1980s, many warnings against the risk cancer following Billroth II reconstruction were published; many authors concluded that bile reflux was related to a higher rate of gastric-stump cancer in patients who underwent Billroth II for benign disease compared with patients who underwent to Billroth I reconstruction. Although not all authors noted this difference, it must be considered that at that time of those early reports, the potential role of *Helicobacter pylori* was not yet understood. Of 827 gastric-stump cancers in patient treated with Billroth I or II for benign disease, Tersmette et al. showed that the difference in cancer rate was not significant between the two procedures [19], and similar concepts were reprised by Bassily et al. [20]. In a recent meta-analysis, Scozzari et al. [8] reported 33 cases of esophageal and gastric cancers after bariatric procedures. Although four (12.1%) cancers appeared after MGB/OAGB, three were detected in the excluded stomach and only one in the gastric pouch, which was following a 1980 surgery that certainly was not a MGB (which was first described in 2001 [2]). On the other hand, the same paper showed 15 cases of esophageal and gastric cancers (45.4%) following restrictive bariatric procedures (LAGB, VBG, SG) and 14 cases (42.4%) after RYGB.

8.5 Conclusions

The MGB/OAGB appears extremely effective in reducing obesity-related comorbidities, offering a good quality of life with a very acceptable complication rate.

References

1. Mason EE, Ito C (1967) Gastric bypass in obesity. Surg Clin North Am 47:1345–1351
2. Rutledge R (2001) The mini-gastric bypass: experience with the first 1,274 cases. Obes Surg 11:276–280

3. Carbajo MA, Garcia-Caballero M, Toledano M et al (2005) One anastomosis gastric bypass by laparoscopy: results of the first 209 patients. Obes Surg 15:398–404
4. Lee WJ, Lin YH (2014) Single-anastomosis gastric bypass (SAGB): appraisal of clinical evidence. Obes Surg 24:1749–1756
5. Chevallier JM, Arman GA, Guenzi M et al (2015) One thousand single anastomosis (omega loop) gastric bypasses to treat morbid obesity in a 7-year period: outcomes show few complications and good efficacy. Obes Surg 25:951–958
6. Musella M, Milone M (2014) Still "controversies" about the mini gastric bypass? Obes Surg 24:643–644
7. Musella M, Susa A, Greco F et al (2014) The laparoscopic mini-gastric bypass: the Italian experience: outcomes from 974 consecutive cases in a multicenter review. Surg Endosc 28:156–163
8. Scozzari G, Trapani R, Toppino M, Morino M (2013) Esophagogastric cancer after bariatric surgery: systematic review of the literature. Surg Obes Relat Dis 9:133–142
9. Bruzzi M, Rau C, Voron T et al (2015) Single anastomosis or mini-gastric bypass: long-term results and quality of life after a 5-year follow-up. Surg Obes Relat Dis 11:321–326
10. Angrisani L, Santonicola A, Iovino P et al (2013) Bariatric surgery worldwide. Obes Surg 25:1822–1832
11. Noun R, Skaff J, Riachi E (2012) One thousand mini-gastric bypass: short and long term outcome. Obes Surg 22:697–703
12. Lee WJ, Wang W (2005) Laparoscopic Roux-en-Y versus mini-gastric bypass for the treatment of morbid obesity: a prospective randomized controlled clinical trial. Ann Surg 242:20–28
13. Lee WJ, Ser KH, Lee YC (2012) Laparoscopic Roux-en-Y versus mini-gastric bypass for the treatment of morbid obesity: a 10-year experience. Obes Surg 22:1827–1834
14. Quan Y, Huang A, Ye M (2015) Efficacy of laparoscopic mini gastric bypass for obesity and type 2 diabetes mellitus: a systematic review and meta-analysis. Gastroenterol Res Pract [Epub ahead of print] doi:10/1155/2015/152852
15. Lee WJ, Wang W, LeeYC et al (2008) Effect of laparoscopic mini-gastric bypass for type 2 diabetes mellitus: comparison of BMI >35 kg/m^2. J Gastrointest Surg 12:945–952
16. Lee Wj, Chong K, Chen CY et al (2011) Diabetes remission and insulin secretion after gastric bypass in patients with body mass index <35 kg/m^2. Obes Surg 21:889–895
17. Musella M, Apers J, Rheinwalt K et al (2015) Efficacy of bariatric surgery in type 2 diabetes mellitus remission: the role of mini gastric bypass/one anastomosis gastric bypass and sleeve gastrectomy at 1 year of follow-up. A European survey. Obes Surg 26:933–940
18. Lee WJ, Wang W, Lee Y (2011) Revisional surgery for laparoscopic mini-gastric bypass. Surg Obes Rel Dis 7:486–492
19. Tersmette AC, Offerhaus GJ, Tersmette KW (1990) Meta-analysis of the risk of gastric stump cancer: detection of high risk patient subsets for stomach cancer after remote partial gastrectomy for benign conditions. Cancer Res 50:6486–6489
20. Bassily R, Smallwood RA, Crotty B (2000) Risk of gastric cancer is not increased after partial gastrectomy. J Gastroenterol Hepatol 15:762–765

Standard Biliopancreatic Diversion

9

Nicola Scopinaro, Giovanni Camerini, and Francesco S. Papadia

9.1   What Do We Mean by Standard Biliopancreatic Diversion?

The issues addressed in this chapter essentially consist of first defining what we mean by "standard" biliopancreatic diversion (BPD). In reality, more than an operation, BPD is a mechanism of action aimed at reducing energy absorption by delaying the meeting between food and biliopancreatic juices. The consequently limited gastrointestinal digestion results in a limited absorption of energy-rich aliments that, if absorbed energy is smaller than total energy expenditure, causes weight loss, which leads to a lower weight of stabilization. This was the main aim when more than 40 years ago, the first author conceived of BPD. The operation is neither difficult nor new, as something very similar had been done before for more than one century for treating peptic disease. A distal gastrectomy is created to minimize the risk of stomal ulcer by using a long Roux-en-Y reconstruction, where the enteroenteroanastomosis (EEA) is placed at a short distance from the ileocecal valve (ICV). The biliopancreatic limb (BPL) coming from the duodenum conveys bile and pancreatic juice to the distal ileum. The stomach, through a wide gastroenterostomy (GEA), empties into the alimentary limb (AL), where all essential aliments can be absorbed. Digestion, and thus fat and starch absorption, is confined to the common limb (CL) after the delayed meeting of food with biliopancreatic secretion.

The CL is then the core of BPD, and all operations involving a CL, where the delayed meeting between food and biliopancreatic secretion occurs, is to be considered a BPD. The degree of intestinal energy malabsorption (current definition of reduced absorption) is determined by the volume of the stomach in-continuity and the length of the intestinal limbs so that any good or bad

N. Scopinaro (✉)
Department of Surgery, University of Genoa Medical School
Genoa, Italy
e-mail: nicola.scopinaro@gmail.com

L. Angrisani (Ed), Bariatric and Metabolic Surgery,
Updates in Surgery
DOI: 10.1007/ 978-88-470-3944-5_9, © Springer-Verlag Italia 2017

result can be obtained by varying the above elements – from the very dangerous distal gastric bypass [1], with small stomach and short CL, to the modern, safe, and effective laparoscopic Roux-en-Y gastric bypass (LRYGB) [2], in which, due to the very long CL, no energy malabsorption occurs. Between these two extremes, hundreds of different BPD with different gastrectomies and different limb lengths exist, including: BPD with preservation of the distal stomach [3] or the entire stomach [4] with pylorus preservation; BPD with sleeve gastrectomy and duodenal switch (BPD-DS) [5]; BPD with vertical instead of horizontal section and pylorus preservation; and the so-called "mini-gastric bypass" [6] – the correct definition of which is "one anastomosis gastric bypass" (OAGB) [7] – which is actually a BPD in which the AL and the BPL coincide and the CL goes from the GEA to the ICV. This is obviously the only small-bowel segment that should be measured, as in the "single anastomosis duodenoileal bypass with sleeve gastrectomy" (SADI-S) [8].

So, what do we mean by "standard BPD"? Some consider it an alternative to BPD-DS, which simply represents the American version of BPD. It conforms to all the rules for BPD, and its results and complications depend on the gastric volume and intestinal limb lengths, exactly as with all other BPD versions, so there is no reason to consider it separately from the latter. Others use the term "standard" to indicate the BPD as performed by the originator. However, the BPD was often modified by its originator in relation to gastric volume and limb length from the time of its conception until a few years ago, with each change entailing different results and complications. Therefore, none of the different models of BPD used during its 30-year evolution could be considered "standard".

The most reasonable solution would be to attribute the term "standard" to the BPD version currently used by the originator, a version that, after 30 years of clinical experimentation accompanied by all pertinent studies has evolved to represent the best compromise between safety and effectiveness. The current model has been used since 2006 (see below), so that despite the 40-year history and evolution of BPD, the "standard BPD" has barely had 10 years of use; its paired results and complications cannot be reasonably given at more than 5 years. For very long-term weight loss results, we usually refer to a group of 40 patients with a minimum follow-up of >30 years and whose BPD model was the so-called "half-half BPD" (HH-BPD), in which the small bowel was cut at its midpoint and the CL was 50-cm in length. Therefore, the operation was rather similar to the one currently used. Weight loss yielded by the HH-BPD was ~70% of the excess, which is not an extraordinarily good result if we consider that the mean initial excess weight of those 40 patients was only 83%. Today, with the current BPD model, we obtain the same percentage of excess weight loss (EW%L) in a population with a mean excess weight >120%. The exciting result was that this 70% of loss was strictly maintained for >30 years, as it was, even over a shorter follow-up period, with all subsequent models of BPD.

Before examining results obtained with the current model of BPD, we believe it is extremely helpful to describe the origin of the operation, its rationale, its physiology, and its evolution over 30 years of unceasing attempts to ameliorate weight loss and reduce surgical complications, until achieving which, as noted above, is the best compromise between effectiveness and safety.

9.2   Origin, Rationale, and Basic Physiology of BPD

Let us start with when, why, and how BPD was developed. In 1972, the first author was 27 years old, and, having begun early as a medical student, he already had an 8-year experience with scientific work, publishing about 20 articles. However, he was looking to pursue a speciality that was really new, at least in Italy.

Everything began when his father, who was Professor of Medicine at the University of Genoa, showed him the 1967 article by Edward Mason on gastric bypass for surgical treatment of obesity [9]. Nobody in Italy had done it before. A few months later, the first author had read everything he could find on that subject, especially on the physiology of intestinal absorption and human nutrition. This research obviously began with the historical article by Kremen et al. [10], in which the first jejunoileal bypass (JIB) was mentioned.

Using a surgical procedure to treat obesity was a very new concept, but if it had been only gastric restriction we would have never made the decision of getting involved with that not even yet born discipline. From both a clinical and scientific point of view, it appeared highly unlikely that it could be the definitive solution to the problem. Much more fascinating and promising was the reduction of intestinal absorption achieved using JIB. We were absolutely convinced that it was the only possible way to obtain complete and definitive solution of the problem, but certainly not with the existing operation, the JIB, which deserved the horrific definition of malabsorption (it could not work that way, it was clear enough without even the need to try it). However, we succeeded in convincing our Professor and Chairman, and in 1973 we performed five JIB according to the Buchwald and Varco technique [11], with poor results. In the mean time we started our experimental study on dogs, which we presented in 1974 [12].

In our first publications [13, 14], we reported the three main defects of the JIB. Finding solutions to these defects was the rationale behind our new operative technique. The presence of a long, excluded loop was an issue, but the unavoidable functional problems of JIB were the indiscriminate malabsorption on one hand and the quick recovery of intestinal energy-absorption capacity on the other. Separating the absorption of beneficial nutrients and that of nonbeneficial energy would allow the resolution of both problems.

On one hand, altering digestion rather than absorption creates a malabsorption that is essentially selective for fat and starch, thus preserving absorption of essential nutrients. On the other hand, selective malabsorption of energy can neutralize the intestinal adaptive phenomena, which cause rapid recovery of the energy-absorption capacity after JIB [15].

We know that if the small bowel in-continuity between the duodenum and ileocecal valve is >60 cm, no substantial weight loss will occur; on the contrary, if it is <40 cm, it is incompatible with life. Realistically, any length between 40 and 60 cm is destined to fail. The why can be found in articles by Dowling [16, 17], who explored in depth the mechanisms and regulation of intestinal adaptation. Intestinal adaptation necessitates both general enterohormonal stimulation, represented by enteroglucagon and neurotensin, and intraluminal stimulus, represented by food and/or biliopancreatic secretion. Both these signals are needed, none of them would work alone. After JIB, the general stimulus remains intact, but the excluded bowel receives no intraluminal signal and becomes hypertrophic, while the small bowel in-continuity receives both food and biliopancreatic juice. It thus undergoes a huge adaptation that results in a more than tenfold increase in energy-absorption capacity, thus totally nullifying the initial malabsorption, with consequent weight regain. We carefully studied all aspects of anatomofunctional adaptive changes following JIB [18, 19], showing very rapid recovery of both fat and starch absorption. Finally, the 1980 article by Halverson et al. [20] definitively killed the JIB, demonstrating that, mainly due to weight regain, only 18% of results could be considered good. Weight regain, not complications, was the main cause of JIB abandonment.

Conversely, after BPD, the entire small bowel receives the intraluminal stimulation from food and/or biliopancreatic secretion, so the entire small bowel goes into hypertrophy [21], although not as greatly as in JIB. However, because it involves the whole small bowel, it accounts for an increase in visceral mass by ~1 kg. The corresponding increase in resting energy expenditure of almost 400 kcal/day plays a very important role in the weight loss that follows BPD [22].

The most important consequence of the separation of energy-rich food absorption and essential nutrient absorption is the possibility of neutralizing the effect of intestinal adaptation. Actually, since the absorption of protein and other essential nutrients occurs in the AL, the CL can be created at any length, including the length that will result exactly in the desired fat absorption capacity after intestinal adaptation. Consequently, after intestinal adaptation, intestinal energy absorption remains constant indefinitely, which explains the durable weight maintenance that follows BPD.

Two years of experimental work on 12 dogs [14, 23] included all the important studies: complete blood and urine biochemistry were done preoperatively and weekly during the first month. Fat absorption as a percentage of intake (modified Kramer's method), protein absorption as a percentage of intake (^{125}I-albumin fecal excretion), and intestinal absorption of bile acid [1-(^{14}C)-glycine-glycocholate fecal excretion] were done preoperatively and at 1, 6, and 12 months. Gallbladder bile composition (bile acid, cholesterol, phospholipid concentration) and wedge liver biopsy were recorded at operation and at sacrifice. Liver function tests were done preoperatively and at 1, 3, 6, and 12 months.

The first human BPD was done on 12 May 1976. Although the patient lost only 40% of excess weight, that loss was consistently maintained for more than 30 years [24].

9.3   Development of BPD

Appropriate intestinal limb length and stomach volume evolved with the progressive information derived from the continuous study of the BPD's physiology and results [25, 26].

The original philosophy for limiting digestion in BPD was to delay the meThe original philosophy for limiting digestion in BPD was to delay the meeting between food and biliopancreatic juice in order to confine pancreatic digestion to a short segment of small bowel. In the first experimental model of BPD (1976), BPL length was only 30 cm and CL was 100 cm, so that the AL was ~6-m long. Protein absorption (see also section 9.5.1) was undisturbed (97.5 ± 5.6%) in these first five patients, but weight loss was unsatisfactory (~40%). We believed that was partly due to the CL being too long and partly to the digestive activity of brush-border enzymes in the AL. In a subsequent model, again five cases, CL length was reduced to 75 cm, while 1–2 m of small bowel were added to BPL length, thus shortening the AL (biliopancreatojejunal diversion type I, or BPJD I). Protein absorption was still nearly complete (94.9 ± 1.8%), and although weight loss was greater, it was not satisfactory (~50%). In the five patients in the third model (BPJD II), we moved the first half of the small bowel in the BPL without varying CL length. Weight loss further increased (~60%) and protein absorption decreased (76.2 ± 11.5; p<0.05 vs. BPD and BPJD I), demonstrating the importance of intestinal enzyme digestion for both starch and protein. At that point, BPL length was sufficient to allow complete digestion-absorption of the scarce (as non meal-stimulated) pancreatic enzymes so that pancreatic digestion no longer occurred in the CL (unpublished experimental data). Consequently, starch and protein absorption depended on the length of small bowel between the GEA and the ICV, while fat absorption, which needs the presence of bile salts, occurred only in the CL. This was proven by the subsequent model, the so-called BPJD III, or half-half (HH-BPD), in which the length of small bowel between GEA and the ICV was unchanged but CL length was shortened to 50 cm. In the 12 patients in that model, protein absorption did not change (77.2 ± 7.3; p<0.01 vs. BPD and BPJD I), while weight loss showed a further increase (~70%), evidently due to the reduced fat absorption. With the subsequent model – the so-called "short-loop BPD", in which the AL was reduced to 2 m – we achieved a further increase in weight loss (~80%) and decrease in protein absorption (~70%), which in some cases caused protein malnutrition (PM). These intestinal lengths were used for a long time (1980–1992), this being our model at the time of our very important study on intestinal energy, fat, and nitrogen absorption [27]. That study confirmed what we had already hypothesized from the very strict weight maintenance that follows BPD, that is, that the BPD digestive-absorptive apparatus has a maximum energy (fat and starch) transport capacity, which corresponds to about 1250 kcal/day, and consequently, all energy intake exceeding the maximum transport threshold is not absorbed. Therefore, since daily energy intake is largely higher than the aforementioned threshold, daily energy absorption remains constant for each patient regardless of energy intake. The same absorption study also revealed the existence of a fivefold increase in endogenous nitrogen loss, which doubles daily protein requirement and is the main cause of PM.

All changes in gastric remnant volume were done in the BPD model with a CL length of 50 cm and AL length 200 cm [22]. In the BPD model currently used, few if any pancreatic enzymes reach the CL, so no pancreatic digestion occurs there. All digestive capacity is in the intestinal brush-border enzymes, so protein and starches are digested and absorbed in the entire intestinal segment between the GEA and the ICV. Due to the necessity of bile salt, only fat absorption is limited to the CL. Therefore, a longer AL means increased protein absorption; however, the concomitant increase in starch absorption reduces weight loss and results in higher stabilization weight.

The other important item in BPD is stomach volume. The smaller its volume, the more rapidly it empties. Along with appetite reduction due to increased production of anorexigenic ileal hormones glucagon-like peptide (GLP-1) and peptide tyrosine-tyrosine (PYY) [28, 29], the rapid gastric emptying that occurs during the first postoperative months causes a more intense postcibal effect, with excessive reduction of food intake and increased risk of early PM. In the later postoperative period, when postcibal syndrome has subsided, it causes quicker intestinal transit and thus reduced energy and protein absorption, resulting in greater weight loss, lower stabilization weight, and an increased risk of recurrent PM. The problem was then to find the best combination of stomach volume, the reduction of which can cause excellent weight loss but a high risk of PM, and AL length, the increase of which makes the operation safer but less effective.

In the early phase of BPD evolution, the impressive weight loss obtained by reducing gastric remnant volume was attractive. However, due to the above-mentioned aspects of BPD physiology in the so-called "very little stomach" model (219 patients; 1982–1983), in which a mean of 150-mL gastric volume was left, a spectacular reduction of 90% of the initial weight resulted in a catastrophic incidence of 30% PM, with 9% being recurrent and was often accompanied by excessive weight loss. The importance of gastric volume was evidenced by the fact that the mean gastric volume of malnourished patients was significantly smaller than that of non-malnourished patients.

At that point, rather than grossly and blindly increasing gastric volume and AL length concomitantly – which would eliminate the problems – we chose to determine the best compromise between effectiveness and safety. In 1984, we began using the "ad hoc stomach-BPD" (AHS-BPD), in which gastric volume is adapted to the individual patient's characteristics [22]. Mean weight loss curve with the AHS-BPD at a minimum follow-up of 5 years clearly showed that the initial percentage of excess weight loss (EW%L) of 80% was reduced to the current 70% while eliminating PM.

The initial aim of AHS-BPD was to confine the risk of PM to patients who required greater weight loss by adapting gastric volume to the initial excess weight only. The mean gastric volume was increased to ~300 mL, with an overall PM incidence of 15% and a still very good %EWL of 79% (first 192 AHS-BPD patients). Obviously, patients with gastric volume <300 mL had still a significantly greater incidence of PM. In 1987, effectiveness was reduced in favor of safety by adapting the gastric volume to other patient characteristics, namely, age, sex, eating habits, and expected degree of compliance. The new rationale was to select only patients with the most likely individual characteristics to take advantage of the risk/benefit of a smaller stomach. Results, in the subsequent 859 AHS-BPD patients, were an 11% overall incidence of PM, with 4.5 recurrence rate and loss of initial excess weight reduced to 74%. At that point, the disappearance of any significant difference in gastric volume between PM and non-PM patients demonstrated that gastric volume had no more influence on PM incidence.

Therefore, in order to further minimize the PM complication, in 1992 we began adapting also the AL length to patients' individual characteristics, with social-behavioral characteristics involved with the risk of PM being protein content of customary food, capacity to modify eating habits according to individual needs, and financial status. Initially (230 patients), AL length was increased to 300 cm in patients at risk. After poor weight loss results in the first 100 patients with a 300-cm AL length (68% loss of initial excess weight), we decreased the maximum AL length to 250 cm. The resulting ad hoc stomach/ad hoc AL BPD (AHS-AHAL-BPD) in the first 300 patients with a minimum follow-up of 10 years resulted in the almost negligible incidence of 1%recurrent PM, reoperations for late specific complications being required in only 1% of patients while maintaining very good permanent reduction of 71% in initial excess weight. The fact that this policy yields the best compromise between effectiveness and safety was confirmed by a BAROS (Bariatric Analysis Reporting Outcome System) evaluation of more than 800 patients [30], which showed that among patients operated on after 1992 there was only a 2% failure rate, with more than 90% of results being from good to excellent.

In 2006, a sufficient number of patients had a minimum follow-up of 10 years to compare results and complications obtained with the three different AL lengths. Since the incidence of PM was negligible in both the 300- and the 250-cm groups and long-term weight loss in the 250-cm group was not significantly different from that of the classic 200-cm length, the 250-cm AL length was used in all subsequent patients, who thus far have maintained very good weight loss with a total absence of PM.

In conclusion, a good knowledge of BPD physiology, together with a very long, careful clinical study, allowed the adaptation of both gastric volume and AL length to the individual patient's characteristics. The resulting revision rate for late specific complications of <1% made BPD during the last 15 years – in our hands and in well-selected patients – not only the most effective but also the safest operation yet available for obesity treatment.

9.4   Results

Weight-loss results have been exhaustively reported above in detail while referring to each subsequent BPD developmental model. The current BPD model, with a mean gastric volume of 400 mL and an AL and CL measuring 250 and 50 cm, respectively, yields a mean reduction of initial excess weight of 70%, strictly maintained up to the fifth postoperative year in the 366 severely obese patients operated on in the years 2006–2011. Mean percent reductions of initial excess weight obtained with each subsequent BPD model, developed during BPD evolution, was rigorously maintained for more than 30 years, irrespective of patient size, weight loss. Therefore, a similar trend is expected with the weight-loss results of the present – and thus far, definitive – model.

The total number of BPD operation performed at our institution from 1976 to the end of 2015 was 3,439. This included 123 patients with BMI <35 kg/m^2 operated on between May 2007 and June 2010. Indication for their surgery was mainly or solely to treat type 2 diabetes mellitus (T2DM).

The other beneficial side effects of BPD are those consequent to weight loss, and, thanks to the characteristics of weight reduction that follows the operation, they are particularly good and they are permanent. Moreover, BPD possesses some specific actions totally independent of weight loss that ensure the very-long-term normalization of serum cholesterol [31, 32] and remission of T2DM in the near totality of these patients [33, 34]. Excellent short-term results were also obtained in T2DM patients with BMI 25–35 kg/m^2 [35–37].

9.5   Complications

BPD has a 2–3% incidence of stomal ulcer, which responds well to medical therapy. Risk is confined to the first 2 postoperative years [22], except in smokers, who may have recurrent stomal ulcers with possible eventual GEA stenosis, which can require a higher gastrectomy.

An important long-term issue with BPD is patient noncompliance with taking lifelong supplementation, namely: Fe, Ca [38, 39], and more importantly, liposoluble vitamins, especially A and E. Deficiency is easily diagnosed and treated in all except vitamin E. Vitamin E deficiency can develop surreptitiously for many years after BPD, and the presenting symptom may be severe neurological problems similar to those that can be caused by early acute thiamine deficiency [40]. We strongly recommend yearly test for serum vitamin levels; however, only the most compliant patient do so. Therefore, since an active lifelong follow-up is substantially impossible with most patients, we drastically reduced the use of BPD in our patient population to only ~20%.

Protein-energy malnutrition (PEM) is a serious complication of BPD that deserves an accurate description regarding pathogenesis, prevention, and treatment, though, due to accurate patients' selection, it has essentially disappeared in our hands.

9.5.1 Protein-Energy Malnutrition after BPD

Protein absorption was studied at the beginning and end of clinical experimentation [41, 42] by measuring fecal radioactivity for 3 days after administration of 10 μC of 125I-albumin with a meal containing 60 g of protein. Both studies demonstrated an alimentary protein absorption rate of ~70% of intake. Since a 30% reduction of protein absorption did not explain the occurrence of PM, we did a more accurate study [27] by directly measuring nitrogen content of food and stools in 15 long-term BPD patients. Comparing alimentary protein absorption, confirmed at 73%, and nitrogen apparent absorption revealed a fivefold increase in endogenous nitrogen loss. This finding raised the daily protein requirement from ~40 to ~90 g/day. This increase does not represent a problem considering that the long-term BPD patients in our study had an average protein intake of ~170 g/day.

Of much greater impact is the endogenous protein loss in the early postoperative period, when the forcedly reduced food intake barely allows protein intake to compensate for the normal protein requirement plus the endogenous extra protein loss. The latter is evidently due to the presence of food in intestinal segments that are not normally in contact with food (ileum and colon). As food intake gradually increases during the early postoperative months, endogenous nitrogen loss and thus protein requirement also progressively increase until the ileal and colonic protein absorption capacities have been completely saturated. At that point, and only at that point, will the protein requirement remain constant. Any further progressive increase in food intake, up to the large amount observed in our long-term study, will gradually reduce the risk of protein nutrition problems. This is then the critical point, as any added form of preventing increased food intake will result in a high risk of PM.

The early postoperative months are the risky period, when the forcedly reduced food intake causes a negative balance of both energy and nitrogen, thus inducing PEM. Depending on the patient's eating behavior, PEM will develop in one of its two classic forms: marasmic or hypoalbuminemic form, the latter being the so-called kwashiorkor [43].

If patients devote the little eating capacity that remains immediately after BPD to mainly protein-rich food, marasmic PEM will develop, which is simply the effective metabolic adaptation to starvation. Both nitrogen and energy deficits are present, and the ensuing hypoinsulinemia allows lipolysis and proteolysis in the skeletal muscle, which is our physiologic protein store. This supplies amino acids for visceral-pool preservation and, through glyconeogenesis, hepatic synthesis of glucose, which is necessary for brain, heart, and kidney metabolism and for fatty acid oxidation. All this, in association with protein and energy sparing due to the negative energy balance, ensures both protein and energy homeostasis. In other words, in marasmic PEM, the organism is in deficit of protein and energy but can draw on its protein and energy stores for homeostasis maintenance. The result is weight loss with harmonic reduction of fat and the fat-free mass in the skeletal muscle only, which is the precise goal of the bariatric operation.

If, conversely, the patient gives preference to carbohydrates, the normal or near-normal energy supply causes hyperinsulinemia, which inhibits both lipolysis and skeletal muscle proteolysis. Not being able to draw on its protein stores, and in absence of protein sparing, the organism reduces visceral protein synthesis, with consequent hypoalbuminemia, edema, anemia, and immunodepression. The result is a severely ill person with body weight unchanged or increased, maintained adipose tissue size, and lean body composition pathologically altered with decreased visceral cell mass and increased extracellular water, which represents the most dangerous nutritional complication of BPD.

Paradoxically, a starving patient is in a better metabolic situation, because the protein store can be drawn upon to satisfy the requirement and compensate for the normal endogenous loss, which obviously is not increased. Furthermore, thanks to lipolysis, the patient can use all the required energy due to neoglycogenesis supplying glucose for the oxidation of fatty acids. This condition, in which the BPD plays no role at all, results in a harmonic weight reduction, such that the patient becomes emaciated, resembling prisoners in the Nazi concentration camps, or, more modernly, children with marasmic PEM in poor African countries. Although in the terminal phase, having lost all or almost all fat and skeletal muscle mass, such individuals remain in a relatively good nutritional status, because their homeostatic visceral proteins are preserved. They eventually die only when all energy sources have been fully exhausted.

Getting back to BPD patients, between the two above-mentioned extreme conditions, hypoalbuminemic PEM of varying severity can take place in patients with mixed intake, depending on how much smaller their protein intake is than their protein requirement plus endogenous protein loss, and how much the relative excess of energy intake prevents skeletal muscle proteolysis, lipolysis, and protein-energy sparing [22].

The pathogenesis of PM after BPD is then multifactorial [44] and depends on certain operation-related variables (gastric volume, intestinal limb lengths, individual capacity of intestinal absorption and adaptation, amount of endogenous protein loss) and on some patient-related variables (customary eating habits, ability to adapt them to the requirements, socioeconomic status). In most cases, PM is limited to a single early episode, with patient-related factor being preeminent. Delayed appearance of sporadic PM is decreasingly frequent as time passes. However, the recurrent form, which is mainly due to operation-related variables, requires surgical revision.

Preventing PM after BPD is essentially based on a good operation and a good patient selection. Since adopting a mean gastric volume of ~400 mL, an AL of 250 cm, and especially the rigorous patient selection according to patient characteristics listed above, we have essentially eliminated the problem at our institution. No more than 20% of our bariatric surgery is now represented by BPD, and the only surgical revisions we are doing are in patients operated on 10 or 20 years ago, or even longer.

Treating early PM in the patient who is still substantially overweight consists of simply converting hypoalbuminemic to marasmic PEM, which allows exploitation of the patient's protein and energy stores. This is easily obtained by annulling alimentary carbohydrate intake, and – taking into account food protein intake – administering intravenously amino acids in amounts sufficient to compensate for the endogenous protein loss. Instead, treating late sporadic PM, when body size is normal or near-normal, must be aimed at eliminating PM and restoring normal nutritional status with parenteral feeding, which includes the nitrogen and energy necessary to restore the amino acid pool, reestablish the anabolic condition, and resynthesize deficient visceral protein.

Detailed knowledge of the different forms of PM pathogenesis is necessary to prevent, diagnose, and treat this most important potential nutritional complication following BPD.

References

1. Liszka T, Sugerman H, Kellum J (1988) Risk/benefit considerations of distal gastric bypass. Int J Obesity Metab Relat Disord 12:604–609
2. Wittgrove AC, Clark GW, Tremblay LJ (1994) Laparoscopic gastric bypass, Roux-en-Y: preliminary report of five cases. Obes Surg 4:353–357
3. Kalfarentzos F, Papadoulas S, Skroubis G et al (2004) Prospective evaluation of biliopancreatic diversion with Roux-en-Y gastric bypass in the super obese. J Gastrointest Surg 8:479–488
4. Vassallo C, Negri L, Della Valle A et al (1997) Biliopancreatic diversion with transitory gastroplasty preserving duodenal bulb: 3 years experience. Obes Surg 7:30–33
5. Hess DS, Hess DW (1998) Biliopancreatic diversion with a duodenal switch. Obes Surg 8:267–282
6. Rutledge R (2001) The mini-gastric bypass: experience with the first 1,274 cases. Obes Surg 11:276–280
7. García-Caballero M, Carbajo M (2004) One anastomosis gastric bypass: a simple, safe and efficient surgical procedure for treating morbid obesity. Nutr Hosp 19:372–375
8. Sánchez-Pernaute A, Herrera MA, Pérez-Aguirre ME et al (2010) Single anastomosis duodeno-ileal bypass with sleeve gastrectomy (SADI-S). One to three-year follow-up. Obes Surg 20:1720–1726
9. Mason EE, Ito C (1967) Gastric bypass in obesity. Surg Clin North Amer 47:1345–1352
10. Kremen AJ, Linner JH, Nelson CH (1954) An experimental evaluation of the nutritional importance of proximal and distal small intestine. Ann Surg 140:439–443
11. Buchvald H, Varco RL (1971) A bypass operation for obese hyperlipidemic patients. Surgery 70:62–70
12. Scopinaro N, Gianetta E, Pandolfo N et al (1976) Il bypass bilio-pancreatico. Proposta e studio sperimentale preliminare di un nuovo tipo di intervento per la terapia chirurgica funzionale dell'obesità. Relazione al Congresso della Sezione Italiana dell'International College of Surgeons (Napoli, 14-15 dicembre 1974). Minerva Chir 31:560–566

13. Scopinaro N (1974) Intervento in "Tavola rotonda su: Trattamento medico-chirurgico della obesità grave". Accad Med 88–89:215–234
14. Scopinaro N, Gianetta E, Berretti B et al (1976) Valutazione sperimentale del bypass bilio-pancreatico: un nuovo intervento per la terapia chirurgica funzionale della grande obesità. Experimental evaluation of the biliopancreatic bypass: a new operation for the functional surgical therapy of morbid obesity. Atti del I Congresso della Società di Ricerche in Chirurgia (Roma, 4–6 dicembre 1975). Il Policlinico - Sez Chirurgica 83:256–262
15. Solhaug JH, Tvete S (1978) Adaptive changes in the small intestine following bypass operation for obesity. A radiological and histological study. Scand J Gastroenterol 13:401–408
16. Dowling RH, Booth CC (1966) Functional compensation after small bowel resection in man. Demonstration by direct measurement. Lancet 2:146–147
17. Dowling RH (1982) Small bowel adaptation and its regulation. Scan J Gastroenterol 74(Suppl):53–74
18. Scopinaro N, Gianetta E, Berretti B, Caponnetto A (1976) Su un caso di obesità grave trattato mediante creazione di corto-circuito digiuno-ileale. Un anno di decorso clinico. Minerva Chir 31:341–359
19. Battezzati M, Bachi V, Scopinaro N (1976) Esperienza di trattamento dell'obesità grave mediante corto-circuito digiuno-ileale. Minerva Chir 31:494–500
20. Halverson JD, Scheff RJ, Gentry K, Alpers DH (1980) Jejunoileal bypass. Late metabolic sequelae and weight gain. Am J Surg 140:347–350
21. Stock-Damgé C, Aprahamian M, Raul F et al (1986) Intestinal adaptation following biliopancreatic bypass. Clin Nutr 5(Suppl):225–231
22. Scopinaro N, Adami GF, Marinari UM et al (1998) Biliopancreatic diversion. World J Surg 9:936–946
23. Scopinaro N, Gianetta E, Civalleri D et al (1979) Biliopancreatic bypass for obesity: I. An experimental study in dogs. Br J Surg 66:613–617
24. Scopinaro N, Gianetta E, Civalleri D et al (1979) Biliopancreatic bypass for obesity: II. Initial experience in man. Br J Surg 66:618–619
25. Scopinaro N, Gianetta E, Civalleri D et al (1980) Two years of clinical experience with biliopancreatic bypass for obesity. Amer J Clin Nutr 33:506–514
26. Scopinaro N, Gianetta E, Friedman D et al (1986) Evolution of biliopancreatic bypass. Proceedings of the First International Symposium on Obesity Surgery. Genoa, Italy, October 1984. Clin Nutr 5(Suppl):137–146
27. Scopinaro N, Marinari GM, Camerini G et al (2000) Energy and nitrogen absorption after biliopancreatic diversion. Obes Surg 10:436–441
28. Borg CM, Le Roux CW, Ghatei MA et al (2007) Biliopancreatic diversion in rats is associated with intestinal hypertrophy and with increased GLP-1, GLP-2 and PYY levels. Obes Surg 17:1193–1198
29. Valverde I1, Puente J, Martín-Duce A et al (2005) Changes in glucagon-like peptide (GLP-1) secretion after biliopancreatic diversion or vertical banded gastroplasty in obese subjects. Obes Surg 15:387–397
30. Marinari GM, Murelli F, Camerini G et al (2004) A 15-year evaluation of biliopancreatic diversion according to the Bariatric Analysis Reporting Outcome System (BAROS). Obes Surg 14:325–328
31. Gianetta E, Friedman D, Adami GF et al (1985) Effects of biliopancreatic bypass on hypercholesterolemia and hypertriglyceridemia. In: Blommer TJ (ed) Proceedings of the Second Annual Meeting of the American Society for Bariatric Surgery, Iowa City, June 13–14. 138–142
32. Montagna G, Gianetta E, Elicio E et al (1987) Plasma lipid and apoprotein pattern in patients with morbid obesity, before and after biliopancreatic bypass. Atheroscl Cardiovasc Dis 3:1069–1074
33. Scopinaro N, Marinari GM, Camerini GB et al (2005) Specific effects of biliopancreatic diversion on the major components of metabolic syndrome: A long-term follow-up study. Diabetes Care 28:2406–2411

34. Scopinaro N, Papadia F, Camerini G et al (2008) A comparison of a personal series of biliopancreatic diversion and literature data on gastric bypass help to explain the mechanisms of action of resolution of type 2 diabetes by the two operations. Obes Surg 18:1035–1038

35. Scopinaro N, Papadia, F, Marinari G et al (2007) Long-term control of type 2 diabetes mellitus and the other major components of the metabolic syndrome after biliopancreatic diversion in patients with BMI <35 kg/m^2. Obes Surg 17:185–192

36. Scopinaro N, Adami, GF, Papadia FS et al (2011) Effects of biliopancreatic diversion on type 2 diabetes in patients with BMI 25 to 35. Ann Surg 253:699–703

37. Astiarraga B, Gastaldelli A, Muscelli E et al (2012) Biliopancreatic diversion in nonobese patients with type 2 diabetes: impact and mechanisms. J Clin Endocrinol Metab 98:2765–2773

38. Compston JE, Vedi S, Gianetta E et al (1984) Bone histomorphometry and vitamin D status after biliopancreatic bypass for obesity. Gastroenterology 87:350–356

39. Compston JE, Vedi S, Watson GJ et al (1986) Metabolic bone disease in patients with biliopancreatic bypass. Clin Nutr 5(Suppl):221–224

40. Primavera A, Schenone A, Simonetti S et al (1987) Neurologic disorders following biliopancreatic diversion. Proceedings of the Third International Symposium on Obesity Surgery, Genoa, September 20–23, 48–49 (abstract)

41. Bonalumi U, Cafiero F, Caponnetto A et al (1981) Protein absorption studies in biliopancreatic bypass patients. Int J Obesity 5:543 (abstract)

42. Friedman D, Caponnetto A, Gianetta E et al (1987) Protein absorption and protein malnutrition after biliopancreatic diversion. Proceedings of the Third International Symposium on Obesity Surgery, Genoa, September 20–23, 50–51 (abstract)

43. McClave SA, Mitoraj TE, Thielmeier KA, Greenburg RA (1992) Differentiating subtypes (hypoalbuminemic vs marasmic) of protein-calorie malnutrition: incidence and clinical significance in a university hospital setting. JPEN 16:337–342

44. Gianetta E, Friedman D, Adami GF et al (1987) Etiological factors of protein malnutrition after biliopancreatic diversion. Gastroenterol Clin North Am 16:503–504

Duodenal Switch

10

Gianfranco Silecchia, Mario Rizzello, and Francesca Abbatini

10.1　Introduction

The biliopancreatic diversion (BPD) described by Scopinaro et al. in 1976 is a malabsorptive bariatric procedure that combines a horizontal gastric resection with the closure of the duodenal stump, a gastroileostomy, and an ileoileostomy to create a 50-cm common channel and a 250-cm alimentary channel. The original procedure included the routine cholecystectomy and appendectomy [1]. The malabsorption involves mainly substrates like fat and starch. The average daily energy intake is thus reduced to ~1750 kcal. Weight loss after BPD is excellent and long lasting (>15 years) [2–5]. The original Scopinaro BPD is associated with a high rate of marginal ulcers (12%), iron-deficiency anemia (40%), bone demineralization (6%), peripheral neuropathy, protein malnutrition (30%), and dumping syndrome. In order to reduce these complications, in 1998, Hess and Hess, and later Marceau et al., proposed modifying the distal gastrectomy with a vertical gastrectomy (sleeve) to preserve integrity of the vagal supply, the antropyloric region, and elongate the common channel from 50 cm to 100 cm [6–8]. Adopting DeMeester et al.'s criteria to treat alkaline reflux [9], those two groups proposed the duodenoileostomy ~2 cm from the pylorus [duodenal switch (DS)]. Lengthening the common channel to 100 cm was introduced to decrease the number of daily bowel movements [6]. The first laparoscopic BPD-DS was performed in 1999 and represents a current standard technique [10].

From the functional viewpoint, BPD-DS is considered a 'hybrid' bariatric procedure that combines the effects of gastric restriction with those of 'moderate' intestinal malabsorption. The restrictive element of BPD-DS comes from the sleeve gastrectomy (150 mL of volume). Preservation of the antropyloric region without altering physiologic gastric emptying leads to better absorption of many

G. Silecchia (✉)
Department of Medico-Surgical Sciences and Biotechnologies, Division of General Surgery and Bariatric Center, Sapienza University of Rome
Latina, Italy
e-mail: gianfranco.silecchia@uniroma1.it

L. Angrisani (Ed), Bariatric and Metabolic Surgery,
Updates in Surgery
DOI: 10.1007/ 978-88-470-3944-5_10, © Springer-Verlag Italia 2017

nutrients (proteins, calcium, iron, vitamin B_{12}) and reduces the incidence of dumping syndrome. The malabsorptive component results from the intestinal bypass, which is characterized by a 250-cm-long alimentary channel and 100-cm-long common channel. The malabsorptive effect results from keeping food away from bile and pancreatic juices until it reaches the common channel, as with the original Scopinaro BPD. This results in a reduction in caloric and food absorption, particularly of lipids, and metabolic changes through modifications of incretin levels.

Buchwald and Angrisani [11, 12] reported that BPD (in all its variants) represents, to date, less than 2% of the bariatric surgeries performed worldwide. In Italy, BPD (in all its variants) represented only 1.2% of the 11,435 bariatric procedures performed during 2015 (0.16% for BPD-DS) [13]. In spite of the excellent long-term results, the use of BPD-DS throughout the bariatric community remains influenced by the technical complexity, higher complication and mortality rates, and increased risk of protein malnutrition compared with other bariatric procedures [14, 15]. However, significant improvements in the perioperative management of laparoscopic BPD-DS have been reported since the first report in 1999. Considering the high morbidity and mortality rates (38% and 6.25%, respectively) after laparoscopic BPD-DS in super-superobese patients [8], in 2001, Gagner [16] introduced the concept of two-step surgery, the rationale behind which is to obtain a significant weight loss in the first 6–12 months after sleeve gastrectomy (SG) (calibrated on an orogastric bougie >48 Fr) and perform the subsequent intestinal bypass surgery with less technical difficulties and lower incidence of complications [17]. The two-step approach has been adopted worldwide to decrease morbidity and mortality rates after laparoscopic BPD-DS (LBPD-DS), reserving the second step only for patients who did not reach significant weight loss and comorbidity control at 12 months. To date, there is no consensus as to the interval of time between the two steps, but the majority of surgeons and the inventor adopted policy of 'watch and see' to identify, according to patient requirements, the best time for the second step. Furthermore, the mini-invasive approach has brought under discussion the routine performance of BPD-DS consensual procedures (cholecystectomy, appendectomy, liver biopsies) described prior to the laparoscopic era.

10.2   Laparoscopic Surgical Personal Technique

The experience of the first period has been published previously [17]. Since the early 2010s, the two-step procedure has been offered to all superobese patients with a body mass index (BMI) >55 kg/m^2. Initally, sleeve volume was larger (150 mL) than the standard sleeve considered as definitive procedure. Today, we offer a sleeve as definitive procedure to all superobese individuals seeking treatment and the second step is planned in selected cases: insufficient weight loss, weight regain, or failure to control comorbidities. The mean interval is 18 months. The rate of superobese patients requiring the second step ranges from 10 to 15% at 3-year follow-up. Again since the early 2010s, 14 cases of second-step surgery have been performed, with no mortality reported. Three patients (21.4%) presented a fistula of the duodenoileostomy, which was successfully managed conservatively using total enteral nutrition plus proton pump inhibitors and antibiotics i.v. The mean percentage of excess weight loss (%EWL) at 12 months was 65% and all cases with a BMI<35 kg/m².

10.2.1 Preparation

A low-residue diet for 2 days before surgery, a thromboembolic prophylaxis (with low-molecular-weight heparin and compressive systems), and an antibiotic prophylaxis are routinely adopted. During the operation, the patient is placed in the French position, the operator stands between the patient's legs; generally, the assistant with the camera is on the operator's right, and the second assistant on the left. The pneumoperitoneum (15 mmHg) can be induced with a Veress needle through the umbilicus. Once the 30° optical system (10-mm trocar) has been inserted and the anatomic ratios and hepatic margin have been assessed, an additional five trocars are placed under direct vision (one 5 mm, four 10 mm) according to the diagram shown in Fig. 10.1. The 3D full high-definition (HD) equipment allows better vision.

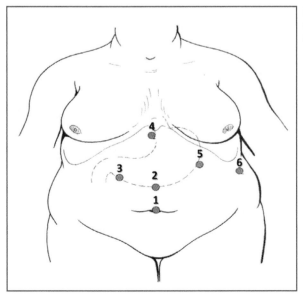

Fig. 10.1 Biliopancreatic diversion–duodenal switch (BPD-DS): trocar placement

10.2.2 Sleeve Gastrectomy (SG)

Our personal technique is described here. Skeletonization of the greater gastric curvature, starting at 6 cm from the pylorus and proceeding upward until the angle of His, is performed using ultrasound dissection (Harmonic Scalpel, Ethicon Endo-Surgery Inc, Cincinnati, OH, USA) or integration of both bipolar and ultrasonic energies (Thunderbeat, Olympus, Japan). Complete exposure of the left crus and the gastroesophageal junction is mandatory. Any hiatal defect, if present, is routinely repaired. The sleeve is created using a linear stapler (Echelon Flex Endopath, Ethicon Endo-Surgery Inc). The stapler is applied next to a 42-Fr bougie placed next to the lesser curve. The stomach is then transected, and a gastric pouch of 80–100 mL is created. Black (4.3 mm) and green (4.1 mm) cartridges are used to transect the antrum, followed by two or three sequential yellow cartridges (3.8 mm) for the gastric body and fundus. In case of revisional SG, only black/green cartridges are used. The staple line is routinely reinforced with Seamguard (W.L. Gore & Associates Inc, Newark, DE, USA). The last cartridge is fired at least 1 cm lateral from the esophagogastric junction in order to preserve vascularization of this critical area. During the vertical dissection, it is important that the assistant carefully retract the stomach laterally to facilitate the proper stapler line without torsion.

10.2.3 Duodenal Sinking

Using an ultrasound dissector or hook coagulator, the pylorus and the first duodenal portion (3–5 cm) are meticulously prepared avoiding vascular or biliary lesions. The duodenum is then divided ~2 cm from the pylorus using a linear stapler with a blue cartridge (3.5 mm) reinforced with buttress material. It might be necessary to complete mobilization of the upper margin of the duodenum as far as the pylorus to facilitate the end-to-side duodenoileal anastomosis.

10.2.4 Ileoileal Anastomosis

The operating table is rotated ~15° to the left. The operator and assistant stand on the patient's left side. Once displayed, the caecum and the distal ileal limb, using an atraumatic grasper marked at 10 cm, the common limb (100 cm), and the alimentary limb (150 cm) are measured. At the latter level, we proceed with the division of the small bowel using a 60-mm linear stapler with white cartridges (2.5 mm). The distal part of the small intestine is anastomosed with the duodenal stump (end-to-side duodenoileal anastomosis), while the proximal part will make up the biliary limb to be anastomosed at the preset distance (100 cm from the ileocecal valve). The side-to-side ileoileal anastomosis defines the common intestinal limb. Placement of approaching stitches [polydioxanone (PDS) 2-0] on the antimesenteric side of the limb facilitates subsequent placement of the linear stapler. After creating two small enterotomies, the jaws of the linear stapler with 60-mm vascular load (2.5 mm) are inserted to accomplish a large anastomosis. The enterotomy is closed with 2-0 PDS barbed sutures.

10.2.5 Duodenoileal Anastomosis

Different methods for creating the duodenoileal anastomosis have been proposed (Fig. 10.2):

- *Hand-Sewen*. Manual suturing, as described by Baltasar [18], is the alternative to the mechanical stapler. End-to-side duodenoileal anastomosis is performed in this case using a continuous manual 2-0 polypropylene suture line in a double layer
- *Side-to-Side*. Side-to-side duodenoileal anastomosis is performed using a linear stapler (30-mm blue cartridge inserted through small enterotomies closed with PDS)
- *End-to-Side*. The inventor of the laparoscopic DS (Gagner) described an end-to-side anastomosis created using a 21-mm circular stapler [10]. We adopted this technique in 2002 [17].

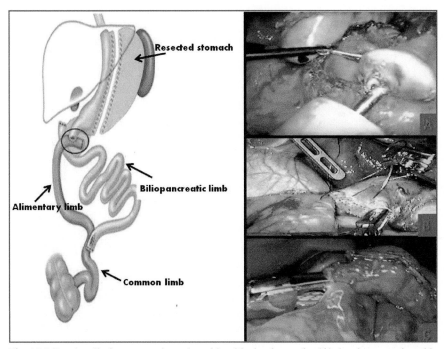

Fig. 10.2 Duodenoileal anastomosis: end-to-side with circular stapler (**A**); hand sewn end-to-side (**B**); side-to-side with linear stapler (**C**)

Placing the anvil of the circular stapler at the duodenal stump can be challenging. Two options are feasible:

a. Considering the eventual difficulties in getting the tube to advance as far the duodenal stump, an anterior antrotomy (anterior wall of the antrum 5 cm from the pylorus) can be carried out to allow direct placement of the anvil in the gastric cavity. The gastrotomy is closed using PDS 2-0. The anvil is introduced into the abdominal cavity using a trocar incision and secured to a stitch to facilitate introduction into the stomach.

b. Transoral placement can be performed using the 21-mm OrVil circular stapler system (3.5 mm) from Medtronic, which was modified to facilitate the proper position of the anvil, including a secure retrieval system in case of anvil disconnection from the orogastric tube.

Currently, we use CEEA Premium Plus 21 mm. During this procedure, the experience and cooperation of a devoted anesthesiologist is crucial. The anesthesiologist inserts the orogastric tube, which has the anvil secured to the tip (DST Series EEA OrVil Devices, Medtronic). A small duodenotomy in the middle portion of the stapler line on the guide of the inserted orogastric tube is created with a monopolar hook, and the tube is retracted in order to advance the anvil through the oropharynx, oesophagus, and the stomach as far as the duodenal stump. The anvil is separated from the tube by cutting the securing stitches and then placed for anastomosis. When using the antecolic route of the small bowel, it is helpful to divide (with ultrasound or radiofrequency dissector) the greater omentum as far as its colonic attachment. Once the anastomosis has been completed, the ileal cul-de-sac is sunk with a 60-mm linear stapler and 2.5-mm blue cartridge.

The procedure is completed with the intraoperative methylene blue test to assess gastric-pouch volume and suture-line integrity. To prevent internal hernias, closure of the mesentery defects with PDS 2-0 is mandatory. Fibrin glue may be placed on both anastomoses. The procedure is completed with the placement of paraanastomotic drainage. It is also recommended to close all 10-mm trocar access sites to prevent trocar-site hernias.

10.2.6 Two-Step Technique

Using four or five trocars, a SG is performed, as described, and the operation ends with the blue methylene test in order assess residual stomach volume. The second step is usually performed 12–18 months later on the basis of patient outcome. At the present, we consider the second step when the patient shows weight regain BMI>35 kg/m^2 with failure of dietician counselling. Recently, our standard policy was changed to offer the second malabsorptive step in selected cases after initial weight loss secondary to SG. Cholecystectomy is indicated only in cases with gallbladder stones.

10.3 Results

10.3.1 Mortality

Thirty-day mortality is low in different experiences. Hess et al. (open BPD-DS), Bolckmans and Himpens (LBPD-DS) and Marceau et al. (open and LBPD-DS) reported a perioperative mortality rate of 0.57%, 0%, 0.76%, and 0.1% respectively [17, 19–22]. The most frequent causes of 30-day mortality following BPD-DS are respiratory complications, especially in patients with obstructive sleep apnea or pulmonary embolism. In the Blockmans and Himpens series, there was a mortality rate of 1.9% (3/153) within 6 months after surgery [20]. After 20 years, Marceau et al. reported a surgery-related mortality rate of 0.57% [21]. There was no mortality in the two-stages LBPD-DS approach used by Silecchia et al. [17].

10.3.2 Weight Loss

With >1400 cases treated since 1988, Hess et al. reported a %EWL of 74% in 148 patients with a 10-year follow-up [19]. Recently, Blockmans and Himpens reported a %EWL of 93% in 113 patients with a 10-year follow-up [20].

Marceau et al. analyzed the influence of common limb (CL) length on weight loss; there was no statistically significant difference between a CL of 75 cm [percentage of excess BMI loss (%EBMIL) 94.4%] and CL of 100 cm (%EBMIL 93.5%). Moreover, there was no statistically significant difference in terms of weight regain between a CL of 75 and 100 cm (28.3% vs. 22.4%; $p=0.49$). When analyzing the outcome in terms of weight loss and regain, superobese participants (BMI>50 kg/m^2) had a significantly better result than the morbidly (not super-) obese (%EBMIL 84 vs. 99%; weight regain 6 vs. 30%).

After a mean long-term follow-up of 9.8 years (2118 patients with >5-year follow-up, 915 with >10-year follow-up) from open BPD-DS, Marceau et al. reported a %EWL of 70.9%, and weight loss was maintained for the whole 20 years [21]. These data provide additional confirmation of the effectiveness of the procedure, which gives long-term results comparable with BPD as regards weight loss.

10.3.3 Revision and Other Operations

In large series with long-term follow-up [20, 21], reoperation for insufficient weight loss ranged from 1.6% to 3.5%; re-sleeve, conversion to distal gastric bypass, and shortening of the common channel are the indicated revision procedures. Denutrition ranged from 1.4% to 10.6%, for which revisional procedures are CL lengthening, conversion to normal anatomy, or feeding jejunostomy. No differences were registered in terms of correlations with CL length (75 vs. 100 cm) and denutrition. Other surgical procedures related to a previous BPD-DS are cholecystectomy, internal hernia repair, incisional hernia repair, surgery for invalidating reflux (hiatoplasty), and adhesiolysis.

10.3.4   Evolution of Comorbidities

Marceau et al. registered a total diabetes remission rate of 93.4%, with resolution of metabolic syndrome in 89% of cases [21]. Blockmans and Himpens reported a rate of complete diabetes remission of 87.5% without de novo or recurring diabetes in a long-term follow-up (>10 years) [20]. In the same series, LDL cholesterol dyslipidemia remission rate ranged from 37% to 95%, hypertriglyceridemia remission rate from 35% to 89.7%, and arterial hypertension remission rate from 60% to 80.9%. However, they also registered an increase of gastroesophageal reflux disease (GERD) from 15% preoperatively to 46.9% postoperatively (43.8% being de novo) [20].

10.3.5   Bowel Habits

In BPD vs. DS analysis, Marceau et al. reported fewer daily bowel movements and less diarrhea, vomiting, and bone pain after DS [21]. Blockmans and Himpens reported 2.3 stools per day and 25.7% of patients with diarrhea (11.5% used medications to control symptoms). When focusing on CL length in connection with bowel habits, no significant differences were reported by the authors. Abdominal bloating was mentioned by 46.9% and disturbing stool odors by 54% [20].

10.4   Complications (According to Clavien-Dindo Classification)

Hess et al. reported a reoperation rate of 3.7% for complications after open BPD-DS [19]. Recently Blockmans and Himpens and Marceau et al. reported an early (<30 days) surgical re-exploration of 10.5% and 3.5% respectively [20, 21]. Moreover, Biertho et al., after 1000 BPD-DS (228 laparoscopic, 772 open) found no differences in terms of total major complications and reoperation rates between laparoscopic and open approaches [22].

On the basis of the published clinical series of BPD-DS, complications can be classified as perioperative (up to 30 days after operation), postoperative (up to 6 months), and late (after 6 months). Based on severity, complications are classified as major or minor (according to Clavien-Dindo grades).

10.4.1 Perioperative and Postoperative Complications

10.4.1.1 Fistula (Grades IIIa–V)

Fistula can involve the gastric suture line after SG, the anastomosis, and the duodenal stump. The incidence of suture-line leak after SG ranges between 0% and 4.6%. Biertho et al. reported no gastric leak after 228 LBPD-DS but registered a 1.9% gastric leak rate after 772 open BPD-DS [22]. Blockmans and Himpens. registered a gastric leak rate of 2.6% for primary procedures and 16.7% for secondary procedures [20]. The critical areas for leak are the proximal third part of the staple line and the transition points between sequential cartridges. To prevent leak, many authors suggest reinforcing the suture line with buttress material, running suture or biological fibrin glue. Anastomotic leak seems to have the same incidence rate in LBPD-DS as in open series (2.5%).

Clinical presentation of the leak involves tachycardia (heart rate >120 beats/minute), hypotension, fever, and abdominal pain. A spiral computed tomography (CT) scan is the most accurate diagnostic tool, especially in cases of low-output fistulas and when there are no signs of hemodynamic instability. The suture line and anastomotic fistulas can be managed successfully by percutaneous drainage plus total parenteral nutrition, gastric acid secretion inhibitors, antibiotics (associated in selected cases with endoscopic endoprosthesis or endoscopic internal drainage) (grade IIIa). In case of large dehiscence with signs of sepsis (grade IV) or failure of conservative management (grade IIIb), the surgical approach may be laparoscopic or open depending on patient status and surgical-team experience. Operative management includes suturing gastric or anastomotic dehiscence, a wide drain with or without creating a jejunostomy in the biliopancreatic limb for decompression, enteral nutrition, and aggressive supportive care.

10.4.1.2 Small-Bowel Obstruction (Grades IIIb, IV)

In their large series (2615 patients), Marceau et al. registered an obstruction rate of 6% after open BPD-DS [21]. Internal hernias are the main cause of intestinal obstruction and are secondary to limb incarceration in mesenteric defect. Blockmans and Himpens reported an incidence of internal and incisional hernia of 8% and 3.5%, respectively [20]. Small-bowel obstruction required surgery in 2.8% vs. the 1.3% reported after open and laparoscopic surgery in Biertho et al.'s experience ($p=0.2$) [22].

Signs and symptoms can be misleading and unspecific (abdominal cramps, nausea, vomiting). Plain abdomen X-rays, upper gastrointestinal (GI) series or spiral CT scan can be diagnostically useful. Surgical management involves adhesiolysis, reduction of herniated loops, and closure of mesenteric defects. Careful closure of the mesenteric defect at the time of operation is the crucial step in preventing this intestinal obstruction.

10.4.1.3 Bleeding (Grades II–IV)

Postoperative bleeding ranges from 1.7% to 10% and seems to be greater following the laparoscopic procedure. However, larger laparoscopic series report a postoperative haemorrhage rate of <3% [21, 22]. Bleeding can be intraluminal (duodenoileal anastomosis, ileoileal anastomosis, SG). Clinically, patients could present with anemia, hypotension, tachycardia, hematemesis, and/or melena. Sometimes, site recognition and relative management represent a challenge. In all cases, management includes serial blood count evaluation and spiral angio-CT scan. Management differs according to bleeding timing. If it occurs in the first postoperative day and is associated with hemodynamic instability, reoperation is recommended. Endoscopy (with adrenaline injection, electrocautery, or endoclips) can be useful. If bleeding occurs after – and furthermore, in the presence of – hemodynamic stability, a conservative approach (fluid administration, blood transfusion when needed) can be adopted. Hand-sewing the duodenoileal anastomosis, using a six-rows vascular load stapler for ileoileal anastomosis, and reinforcement materials over the stapler line have proved to reduce the risk of bleeding.

10.4.1.4 Pulmonary Embolism (Grades II–V)

Pulmonary embolism (PE) is one of the main causes of death in bariatric surgery. The incidence following BPD-DS ranges between 1 and 3% for open procedures and 0.2 and 1% for laparoscopic procedures. In case of PE, the patient presents dyspnea, tachycardia, hypoxemia, hypercapnia, and high D-dimer values. The recommended diagnostic tests are color Doppler ultrasound of the lower limbs and high-resolution pulmonary spiral CT.

10.4.1.5 Anastomotic Ulcer/Stenosis (Grades II, IIIa)

Anastomotic ulcer following BPD is reported in the literature at a percentage between 3 and 10%. Little data are available on incidence rates of duodenal-jejunal anastomotic ulcer and stricture after BPD-DS. In a series of 1000 patients, Biertho et al. reported a bleeding ulcer rate of 0.2% and a stenosis rate of 1% [22]. The laparoscopic approach (especially using circular mechanical stapler) seems to be more frequently associated with these complications. Probably, the routine use of postoperative proton pump inhibitors has considerably contributed to the reduced incidence rate. Clinically, the patient can present with nausea, vomiting, and fullness sensation. Rehospitalization for i.v. therapy and/or endoscopic dilation is advisable.

10.4.2 Late Complications

10.4.2.1 Nutritional Deficiency

Following BPD-DS, duodenal bypass leads to iron-deficiency anemia. In clinical practice, iron and vitamin B_{12} need to be supplemented in order to reduce the risk of anemia. Ileum bypass leads to lipid-soluble nutrient malabsorption (vitamins A, D, E, K). In morbidly obese patients, osteomalacia, secondary to vitamin D dislocation in peripheral fat, ranges between 8 and 30%. After BPD-DS, osteomalacia increases up to 73% and can be symptomatic in 16% of cases despite regular multivitamin supplement consumption. The pathogenesis is caused by malabsorption of calcium and vitamin D. Supplementation with specific preparations is advised. With supplementation, Marceau et al. reported that after 20 years, vitamin B_{12}, folic acid, vitamin D, iron, ferritin, and albumin levels were improved or unchanged from before BPD-DS [21]. Prevalence of deficiencies for all nutritional markers remained below 2%, with no increases over the last 5 years of follow-up. The only measured significant and persistent nutritional marker was an increase, in 22% of patients, of parathyroid hormone (PTH) values, which was correlated with lower calcium levels but not the level of vitamin D. Only in a few cases was supplementation inadequate, due to the lack of adaptation of the small bowel, and reoperation was necessary. Reversing bypass, lengthening the common channel, or feeding jejunostomy is mandatory. Recently, following 1000 BPD-DS procedures, Marceau et al. reported a revisional rate for denutrition of 1% (6.7% when using the Scopinaro BPD) [21].

10.4.2.2 Cholelithiasis (Grades II–IIIb)

Recently Blockmans and Himpens reported a cholecystectomy rate of 9.7% after BPD-DS [20]. For this reason, some authors performed a routine cholecystectomy, even during laparoscopic BPD-DS. However, in 2004, Barbaro et al. recorded a lower incidence of gallstones and cholecystitis in obese patients treated with ursodeoxycholic acid for 6 months after LBPD-DS [23]. Administering 600 mg/day of ursodeoxycholic acid for at least 6 months following surgery is suggested following one- and two-stage procedures. When cholelithiasis is present, it is advisable to perform a cholecystectomy during LBPD-DS [24].

10.5   Conclusions

The excellent long-term weight loss and amelioration of obesity-related diseases after BPD-DS have never been challenged. Buchwald et al. reported that long-term results after BPD-DS are superior to the Roux-en-Y gastric bypass and similar to BPD [11, 14].

BPD-DS is a complex procedure, particularly when performed laparoscopically in superobese patients. This can explain the higher incidence of complications following the laparoscopic compared with the open procedure. However, it has been demonstrated that overall morbidity and mortality rates in high-volume bariatric centers, using postlaparoscopic BPD-DS is similar to open procedure. In high-risk superobese patients, the two stage LBPD-DS seems to be best alternative for reducing mortality, reoperation, and major complication rates.

References

1. Scopinaro N, Gianetta E, Civalleri D et al (1979) Bilio-pancreatic bypass for obesity: II. Initial experience in man. Br J Surg 66:618–620
2. Scopinaro N, Gianetta E, Adami GF et al (1996) Biliopancreatic diversion for obesity at eighteen years. Surgery 119:261–268
3. Scopinaro N, Adami GF, Marinari GM et al (1998) Biliopancreatic diversion. World J Surg 22:933–946
4. Scopinaro N, Marinari GM, Camerini GB et al (2005) Specific effects of biliopancreatic diversion on the major components of metabolic syndrome: a long-term follow-up study. Diabetes Care 28:2406–2411
5. Adami G, Murelli F, Carlini F et al (2005) Long-term effect of biliopancreatic diversion on blood pressure in hypertensive obese patients. Am J Hypertens 18:780–784
6. Hess DS, Hess DW (1998) Biliopancreatic diversion with a duodenal switch. Obes Surg 8:267–282
7. Marceau P, Biron S, Bourque RA et al (1993) Biliopancreatic diversion with a new type of gastrectomy. Obes Surg 3:29–35
8. Marceau P, Hould FS, Simard S et al (1998) Biliopancreatic diversion with duodenal switch. World J Surg 22:947–954
9. DeMeester TR, Fuchs K, Ball C et al (1987) Experimental and clinical results with proximal end-to-end duodenojejunostomy for pathologic duodenogastric reflux. Ann Surg 206:414–426
10. Ren CJ, Patterson E, Gagner M (2000) Laparoscopic biliopancreatic diversion with duodenal switch: a case series of 40 consecutive patients. Obes Surg 10:514–523
11. Buchwald H, Oien D (2009) Metabolic/bariatric surgery worldwide 2008. Obes Surg 19:1605–1611
12. Angrisani L, Santonicola A, Iovino P et al (2015) Bariatric surgery worldwide 2013. Obes Surg 25:1822–1832
13. SICOB - Italian Society of Bariatric and Metabolic Surgery (2016) Indagine conoscitiva: Anno 2015. www.sicob.org/area_04_medici/00_indagine.aspx
14. Buchwald H, Avidor Y, Braunwald E et al (2004) Bariatric surgery: a systematic review and meta-analysis. JAMA 292:1724–1728
15. Topart P, Becouarn G, Ritz P (2012) Comparative early outcomes of three laparoscopic bariatric procedures: sleeve gastrectomy, Roux-en-Y gastric bypass, and biliopancreatic diversion with duodenal switch. Surg Obes Relat Dis 8:250–254
16. Gagner M, Matteotti M (2005) Laparoscopic biliopancreatic diversion with duodenal switch. Surg Clin North Am 85:141-149
17. Silecchia G, Boru C, Pecchia A et al (2006) Effectiveness of laparoscopic sleeve gastrectomy (first stage of biliopancreatic diversion with duodenal switch) on co-morbidities in super-obese high-risk patients. Obes Surg 16:1138–1144
18. Baltasar A (2007) Hand-sewn laparoscopic duodenal switch. Surg Obes Relat Dis 3:94-96
19. Hess DS, Hess DW, Oakley RS (2005) The biliopancreatic diversion with the duodenal switch: results beyond 10 years. Obes Surg 15:408–416
20. Bolckmans R, Himpens J (2016) Long-term (>10 Yrs) outcome of the laparoscopic biliopancreatic diversion with duodenal switch. Ann Surg [Epub ahead of print] doi:10.1097/SLA.0000000000001622

21. Marceau P, Biron S, Marceau S et al (2015) Long-term metabolic outcomes 5 to 20 years after biliopancreatic diversion. Obes Surg 25:1584–1593

22. Biertho L, Lebel S, Marceau S et al (2013) Perioperative complications in a consecutive series of 1000 duodenal switches. Surg Obes Relat Dis 9:63–68

23. Bardaro SJ, Gagner M, Consten E et al (2007) Routine cholecystectomy during laparoscopic biliopancreatic diversion with duodenal switch is not necessary. Surg Obes Relat Dis 3:549-553

24. Sucandy I, Abulfaraj M, Naglak M, Antanavicius G (2016) Risk of biliary events after selective cholecystectomy during biliopancreatic diversion with duodenal switch. Obes Surg 26:531–537

Single Anastomosis Duodenoileal Bypass with Sleeve Gastrectomy

11

Luigi Angrisani, Ariola Hasani, Antonio Vitiello,
Giampaolo Formisano, Antonella Santonicola,
and Michele Lorenzo

11.1   Introduction

The continuous research in the bariatric surgical field aims to offer more effective, less invasive, simpler, and safer procedures in order to face the global challenge of the obesity epidemic. As already occurred with the mini-gastric bypass or one anastomosis gastric bypass, single anastomosis duodenoileal bypass with sleeve gastrectomy is basically a one anastomosis biliopancreatic diversion (BPD)-duodenal switch (DS) procedure and represents another alternative in the armamentarium of the bariatric surgeon.

As often occurs with novel procedures, the nomenclature is not yet standardized: it is defined according to different authors as single anastomosis ileal bypass, loop duodenal switch, mini-DS, duodenoenteric omega switch, stomach intestinal pylorus-sparing (SIPS) surgery. With some differences in gastric tube size and intestinal bypass length, the principle is the same: it is less demanding and eliminate the Roux limb and can potentially reduce postoperative complications without losing metabolic effectiveness of the BPD-DS [1–4].

The BPD was introduced by Scopinaro et al. in 1976 and consisted of a distal gastrectomy with a long Roux-en-Y reconstruction in which the enteroenterostomy is placed at a distal ileal level, namely, 50 cm from the ileocecal valve [5]. The Scopinaro procedure was modified in 1988 by Hess et al. into the BPD-DS. They proposed a vertical gastrectomy along the greater curvature to preserve the integrity of the antropyloric region, as well as a modification of the length of the common channel to 100 cm [6].

The major obstacles of BPD-DS are its technical complexity, complication rates, and possibility of long-term nutritional issues. Nevertheless, BPD and

A. Hasani (✉)
Department of Clinical Medicine and Surgery, University of Naples Federico II
Naples, Italy
e-mail: ariolahasani@libero.it

L. Angrisani (Ed), Bariatric and Metabolic Surgery,
Updates in Surgery
DOI: 10.1007/ 978-88-470-3944-5_11, © Springer-Verlag Italia 2017

BPD-DS are actually considered among the best options for selected morbidly obese patients with associated diseases. In an attempt to simplify such an effective procedure and preserve its principles, the single anastomosis duodenoileal bypass with sleeve gastrectomy (SADI-S) was first described in 2007 by Sánchez-Pernaute and Torres [7]. SADI-S compared with DS eliminates the Roux-en-Y gastric bypass by creating an omega loop, and because of pylorus preservation, bile diversion is unnecessary as the natural barrier remains in place. Preservation of the pylorus provides control of solid stool emptying, reducing the chances of dumping syndrome and assisting in the maintenance of a physiologically based rate of gastric emptying [4]. The immediate benefit is of the need for only one anastomosis, thus saving operative time and potentially reducing postoperative complications. Moreover, since it does not require a mesenteric opening, there is a reduced risk of internal hernia.

SADI-S is a solution to determining a decrease in the postoperative and nutritional effects of BPD-DS while maintaining weight and metabolic benefits linked to fundus resection, pylorus preservation, duodenal exclusion, ileal brake effect, and fat malabsorption [8, 9]. It also represents a valid option for revisional surgery after failed sleeve gastrectomy (SG). With SADI, the malabsorptive component is added to an essentially restrictive procedure, as the DS is the natural complement to SG for improving weight loss outcomes and sustainability. There is no consensus as to the best revisional procedure after failed SG for poor weight loss. When there is evidence of dilation of the sleeve construction, SADI may also be performed with a concomitant resleeve gastrectomy [10–13]. Moreover, SADIS-S is a versatile procedure. According to patient characteristics and surgeon preference, it can be performed with a narrow gastric pouch and a long common channel (300 or 350 cm) or simply remain a malabsorptive procedure with a short common channel (200 or 250 cm) and a wider gastric pouch. However, to date, few data are available in the literature; long-term results (>10 years) and randomized trials are expected.

11.2   Surgical Technique

The patient begins a semiliquid diet the day before the operation. Low-molecular-weight heparin is administered according to body weight in single daily subcutaneous doses, beginning the day before the operation and continuing for at least 15 days. After induction of general anesthesia, the patient is placed supine in a modified lithotomy position with legs abducted and positioned in adjustable stirrups. Preparation is concluded by insertion of a Foley catheter and a gastric tube. A body warmer and an intermittent compression device for deep venous thrombosis prophylaxis are applied. Antibiotics are injected according to the guidelines.

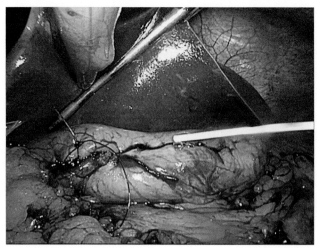

Fig. 11.1 Final aspect of the gastric resection (sleeve)

The surgeon stands between the patient's legs, the camera assistant on the patient's right, and the first assistant on the patient's left. The scrub nurse stands at the lower left side of the table. The pneumoperitoneum is established via a Veress needle at Palmer's point. Trocars are placed as follows: a 10- to 12-mm camera trocar is placed ~20 cm below the xiphoid process a few centimeters left of paramedian; a 5-mm trocar is placed in the subxiphoid area for liver retraction; a 5-mm trocar is placed on the left anterior axillary line; a 10- to 12-mm trocar is placed on the right anterior axillary line; an additional 10- to 12-mm trocar is placed in the umbilicus.

Devascularization of the greater curvature of the stomach is performed with the ultrasonic scalpel (Harmonic, Ethicon Endosurgery, Cincinnati, OH, USA) from the pylorus to the angle of His. The sleeve is then calibrated over a 54-Fr orogastric bougie and the stomach transected with a linear stapler (iDrive Ultra Powered Stapling System, Covidien, Norwalk, CT, USA, or Echelon Flex Endopath Staplers, Ethicon Endosurgery) 60-mm black/green cartridge, starting 3–4 cm from the pylorus. A running introflecting polydioxanone (PDS) 3-0 suture is generally performed to reinforce the staple line (Fig. 11.1). The suture line can also be reinforced by using reinforcement patches like Seamguard or Peri-Strip. Dissection then continues through the first portion of the duodenum down to the gastroduodenal artery. The duodenum is divided with a linear stapler (purple/blue cartridge), preserving vascularization of the lesser curvature (Fig. 11.2).

The patient is placed, at this point, in a horizontal position and the surgeon moves to the left side of the patient. The ileocecal valve is identified and 250 cm are measured upward. The small bowel loop is ascended antecolically and a double-layer continuous handsewn isoperistaltic end-to-side duodenoileal anastomosis is fashioned (Fig. 11.3). The anastomosis is tested for watertightness

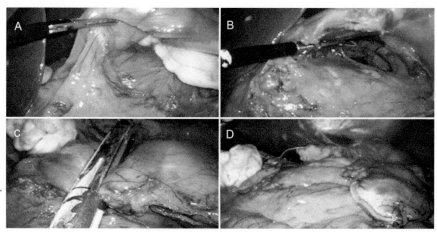

Fig. 11.2 Duodenal dissection. Opening of the lesser sac through swab dissection (**A**, **B**); duodenal transection with a linear stapler (**C**); final aspect after transection, with the proximal duodenum on the right and the duodenal stump on the left (**D**)

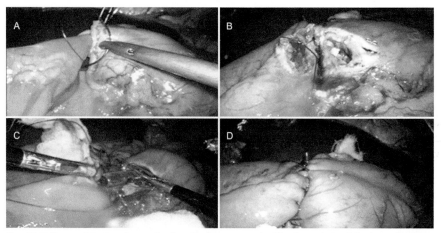

Fig. 11.3 Steps of the handsewn duodenoileal anastomosis. The first stitch of the posterior layer (**A**); aspect of posterior layer of the anastomosis (**B**); introduction of the nasogastric tube through the anastomosis (**C**); final aspect of the handsewn anastomosis (**D**)

by methylene blue instillation orally and covered with fibrin glue, with two bowel clamps in place. The resected stomach is removed through an enlarged port and a suction drain is left in.

When SADI is performed as revision after failed SG, it is necessary to evaluate preoperatively the eventual dilation of the sleeved stomach and the potential need to perform a resleeve. After exploration and evaluation of the sleeved stomach, the procedure starts with the duodenal dissection and preparation, followed by duodenal transection and duodenoileal anastomosis, either performed mechanically or manually.

11.3 Outcomes

When analyzing outcomes of a relatively new procedure, it must first be stressed that few studies are available, no long-term results can be discussed, nomenclature is not yet standardized as well as the common channel length [200 cm vs. 250 cm vs. 300 cm vs. 350 cm, according to different studies and patient's preoperative body mass index (BMI)].

Most of the available studies have been published by Sánchez-Pernaute et al. from Spain. Weight loss has been excellent in these first 3 years, approximating 100% of patients after the first postoperative year. Initial weight loss is even greater than after a classic BPD-DS, which is probably correlated with a potent ileal brake mediated by an enhanced secretion of peptide tyrosine-tyrosine (PYY) and glucagon-like peptide-1 (GLP-1), which stimulate early satiety [9]. An updated report was published by the same group in 2013 on the first 100 patients, who had a mean percentage of excess weight loss (%EWL) of 95%, which was maintained during the follow-up period. However, 3-year results were available only for 19 of the 20 eligible patients.

Moreover, Sánchez-Pernaute et al. recently demonstrated the efficacy of SADI-S in a subgroup of obese diabetic patients and in revisional surgery for patients who experienced weight regain after SG as a stand-alone procedure [10]. Control of the disease, with glycolated hemoglobin (HbA1c) <6%, was obtained in 70–84% in the long term, depending on the initial antidiabetic therapy, with most patients being able to abandon antidiabetic therapy after the operation. An 8% recurrence rate in the first 5 years was registered among the 25 of 32 patients eligible for long-term follow-up [14]. As far as revisional surgery after failed SG is concerned, the authors reported outcomes on 16 patients with an initial BMI of 56.4 kg/m² and a mean %EWL of 39.5% after a SG who underwent SADI with a 250-cm common channel. Their results demonstrated good definitive weight loss after the second procedure, increasing from an initial %EWL of 39.5% to a final 72% after the duodenal bypass, with all patients losing >50% of their initial excess weight. The authors concluded that the loop switch can be considered as a suitable and simplified alternative to BPD-DS after failed SG.

Unpublished data from Mitzman et al. in their series of SIPS – which differs from SADI-S in the size of the orogastric bougie (42 Fr vs. 54 Fr) and in the length of the common channel (300 cm vs. 250 cm) – reported good weight loss outcomes, reaching a mean %EWL of 72.3% after 1 year. The authors believe that preserving 300 cm of intestine along with the ileocecal valve may reduce the risk of malnutrition and diarrhea, and pylorus preservation may assist in maintaining a physiologically based rate of gastric emptying, thus providing an efficacious procedure that offers improved quality of life, reduction in hunger, and increase in satiety while minimizing diarrhea and bowel movements [4].

Recently, an 18-month matched cohort analysis of single anastomosis loop duodenal switch vs. Roux-en-Y gastric bypass was published by Cottam et al. in which 54 patients who underwent RYGB were matched for sex and BMI with 54 patients who underwent SADI-S with a 300-cm-long common channel. SADI-S produced similar but longer-sustained weight loss compared with RYGB, with a reduced variability among patients, as demonstrated by the smaller confidence intervals in their series. It also resulted in fewer complaints of nausea or other upper-gastrointestinal (GI) complaints, with no anastomotic ulcers, resulting in a lower rate of postoperative endoscopies when compared with the RYGB [15].

11.4   Complications (According to Clavien-Dindo Classification)

All bariatric procedures have inherent complications, but while mortality is an easily quantifiable outcome parameter, overall morbidity and its severity are poorly defined. The Clavien-Dindo Classification allows objective quantitation of procedure safety [16]. Short-term postoperative complications include the whole spectrum of events that may occur after a general or bariatric surgery procedures, including leakage/fistula, bleeding, stenosis, and abdominal wall complications.

11.4.1 Leakage (Grade II if Treated Conservatively, Grade IIIb if Treated Endoscopically or Surgically)

Leakage (0.5–2%) can involve the gastric suture line after SG, the anastomosis, and the duodenal stump. Clinical presentation is tachycardia, fever, abdominal pain, and hypotension. An upper-GI X-ray with gastrografin can be useful for diagnosis, but spiral angio-CT scan is the most accurate diagnostic tool. Management can be conservative in case of low-output fistulas (nasogastric tube, percutaneous drainage of fluid collections, total parenteral nutrition). If conservative treatment fails or there is hemodynamic instability and signs of peritonitis, a laparoscopic or laparotomic reoperation is indicated.

11.4.2 Bleeding (Grade II if Treated Conservatively, Grade IIIb if Treated Endoscopically or Surgically)

Bleeding (2%) can be intraluminal (SG, duodenoileal anastomosis) or extraluminal. Clinical presentation is generally clear and characterized by hypotension, tachycardia, anemia, hematemesis, and melena, but identifying the site of and managing it represents a challenge. If the bleeding occurs in the early postoperative period and is associated with hemodynamic instability, a laparoscopic or laparotomic reoperation is indicated. In hemodynamic stability, we adopt a conservative approach (administration of fluids and blood transfusions).

11.4.3 Stenosis (Grades IIIa, IIIb)

No cases of stenosis of the gastric tube or duodenoileal anastomosis have been reported in the published series of SADI-S. One reason is the relatively wide SG, which is calibrated on a larger orogastric bougie (54 Fr).

11.4.4 Abdominal-Wall Complications (Grades I–IIIb)

Abdominal-wall complications are relatively frequent (1–4%).

Surgical-wound infections can occur after bariatric surgery, and they generally require specific antibiotic treatment. Trocar-site hernia, reported in 2% of cases after SADI-S, require surgical correction; this complication may be prevented by carefully closing the trocar sites under laparoscopic view.

11.5   SADI-S and Single-Loop Reconstruction Compared with BPD-DS

The aim of SADI-S is simplifying BPD-DS and reducing its complication rate. At least theoretically, the lack of entero-entero anastomosis alone with SADI-S reduces the anastomotic leak rate. Anastomotic ulcers, reported after BPD, have not been described after SADI-S.

11.5.1 Small-Bowel Obstruction and Internal Hernia (Grade IIIb)

Interestingly, retrograde filling of the afferent limb after SADI-S was reported by Cottam and colleagues. in two patients in whom it caused chronic nausea and partial small-bowel obstruction. After exploratory laparotomy, scar tissue and adhesions were found around the duodenoileal anastomosis, which pulled the efferent limb superior to the anastomosis itself, causing food to enter the afferent limb and symptoms manifesting as partial bowel obstruction. Although this type of procedure is considered to reduce almost to nil the risk of internal hernia, there is a case described by Cottam and colleagues. in which the duodenal ileostomy had scarred and twisted 180 degrees counterclockwise. This caused rolling of the entire afferent limb underneath the anastomosis and over to the right side of the abdominal cavity, creating a partial bowel obstruction [17, 18].

11.5.2 **Protein Malnutrition** (Grade II if Treated Conservatively, Grade IIIb if Treated Endoscopically or Surgically)

Protein malnutrition (0.5-3%) is the most serious complication of SADI-S, as with any BPD. A sustained and rapid weight loss is invariably accompanied by nutritional changes, which reflect the metabolic transformation of the organism. Nutritional changes are characterized by hypoalbuminemia, anemia, asthenia, edema, and alopecia. The pathogenesis of protein malnutrition is multifactorial, being conditioned by some variables linked to the procedure (e.g., gastric volume, intestinal lengths, individual digestion, proteic absorption capacity, amount of lost endogenous nitrogen) and others linked to the patient, such as eating habits and socioeconomic status. Protein malnutrition is generally limited to a single episode during the first postoperative year and is often determined by inadequate eating habits. In case of recurrent hypoalbuminemia, revisional surgery may be necessary. As reported by Sánchez-Pernaute, in these cases, SADI-S is converted to Roux-en-Y duodenal switch with a 300-cm alimentary limb and a 200- to 250-cm common channel by dividing the bowel in the efferent loop just distal to the duodenoileostomy and bringing this end to the biliopancreatic limb 100 cm proximal to the duodenoileostomy [9]. Lifelong follow-up of nutritional status and supplementation are mandatory.

11.6   Conclusions

SADI-S is one of the most recent innovations in bariatric surgery. It represents the continuous research and evolution in this field in an attempt to find more effective and safer solutions when treating the obesity epidemic and metabolic-related diseases. Though no single operation has been demonstrated to date to be the unique solution for all patients with morbid obesity and severe metabolic disease, preliminary results have shown that SADI-S, which is based on the solid physiopathologic principles of BPD-DS, could potentially be a suitable alternative for supermorbidly obese patients.

Standardization of nomenclature and technique, together with further studies with long-term outcomes, are needed to confirm the safety and efficacy of SADI-S in the routine surgical management of the obese population.

References

1. Karcz WK, Kuesters S, Marjanovic G, Grueneberger JM (2013) Duodeno–enteral omega switches—more physiological techniques in metabolic surgery. Wideochir Inne Tech Maloinwazyjne 8:273–279
2. Lee WJ1, Lee KT, Kasama K et al (2014) Laparoscopic single-anastomosis duodenal-jejunal bypass with sleeve gastrectomy (SADJB-SG): short-term result and comparison with gastric bypass. Obes Surg 24:109–113
3. Zaveri H, Surve A, Cottam D et al (2015) Stomach intestinal pylorus sparing surgery (SIPS) with laparoscopic fundoplication (LF): a new approach to gastroesophageal reflux disease (GERD) in the setting of morbid obesity. Springerplus 4:596
4. Mitzman B, Cottam D, Goriparthi R et al (2016) Stomach intestinal pylorus sparing (SIPS) surgery for morbid obesity: retrospective analyses of our preliminary experience. Obes Surg [Epub ahead of print] doi:10.1186/s40064
5. Scopinaro N, Gianetta E, Civalleri D et al (1979) Bilio-pancreatic bypass for obesity: II. Initial experience in man. Br J Surg 66:618–620
6. Hess DS, Hess DW (1998) Biliopancreatic diversion with a duodenal switch. Obes Surg 8:267–282
7. Sánchez-Pernaute A, Rubio Herrera MA, Pérez-Aguirre E et al (2007) Proximal duodenal-ileal end-to-side bypass with sleeve gastrectomy: proposed technique. Obes Surg 17:1614–1618
8. Sánchez-Pernaute A, Rubio MÁ, Pérez Aguirre E et al (2013) Single-anastomosis duodenoileal bypass with sleeve gastrectomy: metabolic improvement and weight loss in first 100 patients. Surg Obes Relat Dis 9:731–735
9. Sánchez-Pernaute A, Herrera MA, Pérez-Aguirre ME et al (2010) Single anastomosis duodenoileal bypass with sleeve gastrectomy (SADI-S). One- to three-year follow-up. Obes Surg 20:1720–1726
10. Sánchez-Pernaute A, Rubio MÁ, Conde M et al (2015) Single-anastomosis duodenoileal bypass as a second step after sleeve gastrectomy. Surg Obes Relat Dis 11:351–355
11. Gagner M, Rogula T (2003) Laparoscopic reoperative sleeve gastrectomy for poor weight loss after biliopancreatic diversion with duodenal switch. Obes Surg 13:649–654
12. Baltasar A, Serra C, Pérez N et al (2006) Re-sleeve gastrectomy. Obes Surg 16:1535–1538
13. Dapri G, Cadière GB, Himpens J (2011) Laparoscopic repeat sleeve gastrectomy versus duodenal switch after isolated sleeve gastrectomy for obesity. Surg Obes Relat Dis 7:38–44
14. Sánchez-Pernaute A, Rubio MÁ, Cabrerizo L et al (2015) Single-anastomosis duodenoileal bypass with sleeve gastrectomy (SADI-S) for obese diabetic patients. Surg Obes Relat Dis 11:1092–1098
15. Cottam A, Cottam D, Medlin W et al (2015) A matched cohort analysis of single anastomosis loop duodenal switch versus Roux-en-Y gastric bypass with 18-month follow-up. Surg Endosc [Epub ahead of print] doi:10.1007/s00464-015-4707-7
16. Goitein D, Raziel A, Szold A, Sakran N (2016) Assessment of perioperative complications following primary bariatric surgery according to the Clavien-Dindo classification: comparison of sleeve gastrectomy and Roux-Y gastric bypass. Surg Endosc 30:273–278
17. Surve A, Zaveri H, Cottam D (2016) Retrograde filling of the afferent limb as a cause of chronic nausea after single anastomosis loop duodenal switch. Surg Obes Relat Dis [Epub ahead of print] doi:10.1016/j.soard.2016.01.018
18. Summerhays C, Cottam D, Cottam A (2016) Internal hernia after revisional laparoscopic loop duodenal switch surgery. Surg Obes Relat Dis 12:e13–e15

Ileal Interposition

12

Diego Foschi, Andrea Rizzi, and Igor Tubazio

12.1 Introduction

In the early 1980s, Koopmans and colleagues [1] first proposed the ileal interposition (II) between the duodenum and jejunum as an experimental surgical procedure to induce reduction of body weight in rodents and dogs. In 1999, Mason [2] considered the increase in enteroglucagon (glucagon-like peptide-1) to be the mechanism of action of II and recommended clinical controlled trials to assess its ability to treat type 2 diabetes mellitus (T2DM) and obesity in humans. In 2006, De Paula et al. [3] described a short series of pathologically obese patients treated by II in association with sleeve gastrectomy (SG) that showed very good results for weight loss and resolution of obesity complications. Several clinical trials investigated the effects of SG with ileal interposition to treat obese patients affected by T2DM or metabolic syndrome (MS). The operation can be performed with diversion of the duodenum (SG-DD-II) or not. In our experience, SG-DD-II is very effective as a bariatric and metabolic operation, although it is highly demanding and needs further evaluation before it will be considered for routine clinical use.

12.2 Experimental Background of Ileal Interposition

The gastrointestinal tract has many intrinsic feedback mechanisms to control secretory, motor, and hormonal functions. As a rule, the distal tract of the intestine is able to regulate activity of the proximal tract by means of hormonal changes [4–6]. Gastric secretion is regulated by the balance between gastrin and somatostatin in the antral mucosa, but several hormones produced by duodenal mucosa [gastric inhibitory peptide (GIP), cholecystokinin (CCK), and intestinal

D. Foschi (✉)
Department of Biomedical Sciences Luigi Sacco, University of Milan
Milan, Italy
e-mail: diego.foschi@unimi.it

L. Angrisani (Ed), Bariatric and Metabolic Surgery,
Updates in Surgery
DOI: 10.1007/ 978-88-470-3944-5_12, © Springer-Verlag Italia 2017

mucosa [glucagon-like peptide 1 and 2 (GLP-1 and -2)] are able to inhibit it. GIP, CCK, and GLP are released by nutrient challenge from endocrine cells. GIP is also known as a glucose-dependent insulinotropic peptide and stimulates insulin secretion; the same effect is exerted by GLP-1 and peptide tyrosine-tyrosine (PYY). These hormones, as well as CCK, pancreatic peptide (PP), and oxyntomodulin also exert anorectic effects and help control food intake and body weight. GIP, GLP-1 and -2, and PYY inhibit gastric emptying and contribute to the regulation of gastrointestinal motility [6]. In the past, short-bowel syndrome was treated by ileal interposition, which makes transit time longer. This effect is mediated by GLP-1 secretion [7]. Furthermore, II reduces food intake and decreases body weight [1] by the same mechanism. Since GLP-1 has a strong incretin effect, II was found to improve glucose and lipid metabolism, delay diabetes onset, and even cure it in experimental animals [7, 8]. From these results, II was considered to be more effective than other operations for curing T2DM in obese patients. However, De Paula (personal communication) found that II alone was not really effective and proposed an association between SG and II [3].

12.3   Indications to Ileal Interposition Surgery

SG-II includes the restrictive effects of SG and the functional effects of ileal interposition, which causes changes in lipid absorption and enterokine secretion. After II, the interposed ileum is unable to absorb fats (because bile salts are released distally in the jejunum) and is rapidly stimulated by chyme to release GLP-1 and -2, fibroblast growth factor-19 (FGF-19), and other hormones that reduce appetite and stimulate insulin secretion. SG-II is indicated mainly for morbidly obese patients with obesity complications [9]. When the duodenum is diverted (SG-DD-II), the operation is highly indicated for treating morbidly obese or obese patients affected by T2DM or MS [10–12]. Moreover, SG with a large remnant or a fundectomy [13] can be associated with II for T2DM patients with a low (<30 kg/m^2) body mass index (BMI) to avoid excessive reduction of body weight [14, 15].

12.4   Surgical Technique

The operation can be performed in two different ways: with or without duodenal diversion [14]. Excluding the duodenum and upper part of the jejunum makes it easier to control glucose homeostasis and allows better results in obese patients with T2DM. We describe SG-DD-II as the standard procedure (Fig. 12.1).

   The operation is performed under general anesthesia as a laparoscopic procedure [3]. Preoperative preparation includes overnight fasting, preoperative

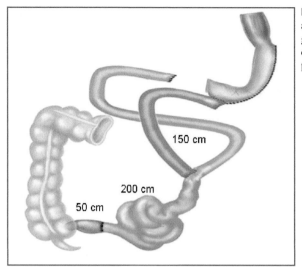

Fig. 12.1 Ileal interposition associated to sleeve gastrectomy and duodenal diversion (reproduced with permission from [16])

bowel cleansing, perioperative antibiotics, and low-molecular-weight heparin prophylaxis. A gastric tube and a urinary catheter are inserted. Seven trocars are used. At the beginning of the operation, the first surgeon is situated between the legs of the patient, who is in an extreme anti-Trendelenburg position. The operation starts with SG after devascularization of the greater curvature of the stomach 6-8 cm from the pylorus, which is achieved using an ultrasonic scalpel. A 36-Fr orogastric calibration tube is placed along the lesser curvature of the stomach toward the pylorus. Gastric resection is performed starting from the antrum and continuing up to the angle of His using an Echelon 60-mm stapler, with gold cartridges in the antrum and blue cartridges in the body of the stomach. Bleeding from the suture line is stopped by bipolar coagulation, but a 3-0 polypropylene running invaginating suture is used in selected cases. After that, dissection of the antrum and duodenum is done with ligature of the right gastric vessels. Duodenum sectioning is performed 4 cm from the pylorus using a linear blue or white cartridge staple. Opening a window in the mesocolon just above the Treitz ligament allows transposition of the stomach and duodenum in the lower abdomen. The stomach is sutured to the mesocolon to avoid internal hernia.

The second step is submesocolic and is performed from the left size of the patient. Measurement of the total intestinal length is performed with traction, along the anti-mesenteric border, using a 5-cm marked atraumatic grasper. In the technique described by De Paula et al. [9], the first transection is done 30 cm from the ileocecal valve; we prefer to maintain 50 cm of distal ileum to reduce the risk of biliary malabsorption. Then, an ileal tract 150- to 170-cm long (50 cm in the first description of De Paula [3]) is prepared using a linear stapler (white cartridge). The interposed ileum is anastomosed to the duodenum. We prefer a gastroileal anastomosis, especially when the duodenum is poorly perfused (Fig. 12.1). A distal anastomosis is done with the jejunum. Finally, the intestinal circuit is restored by suturing the distal jejunum to the distal ileum. In our technique, total intestinal tract length is 400 cm, with a 150-cm transposed ileum (alimentary loop), 250-cm common tract, and a variable pancreatic-biliary tract. The gastroileal anastomosis is performed using a 45-mm linear (blue cartridge) stapler, intestinal anastomoses are performed functionally using 45-mm linear (white cartridge) staplers. The enterotomy defects are closed with a 2-0 absorbable running suture. Mesenteric defects are closed using a continuous 3-0 polypropylene suture line. An abdominal tube is placed in the proximity of the inferior tract of the gastric-line suture.

12.5 Postoperative Course and Complications (According to Clavien-Dindo Classification)

De Paula et al. [9] reported a mean operation time (OT) of 188 min (range 125–330 min) and a median hospital stay (HS) of 3.3. days (range 3-63 days). Higher values [OT 3.9 hours (3.1–8.2), HS 6.9 days (4–429] were reported by Celik et al. [13]. Our mean OT was 290 min (180–480 min), with a mean HS of 8 days (5–60 days). Mortality after SG-DD-II was low (from 0.27 to 0.4%); in all cases, it was caused by septic complications associated with anastomotic leakage. One patient died from myocardial infarction after suture-line leakage of the SG (Clavien-Dindo [17] grade V). The overall rate of major postoperative complications was low: from 4% in the series of De Paula et al. [9] to 6.1% in the series of Celik et al. [13]. We had three cases out of 64 patients: two with leakage and one with bleeding, all of whom required reoperation (Clavien-Dindo grade IIIb). Minor complications were rare: there were three cases of wound infection and wound hematoma (Clavien-Dindo grade I). Constipation and anorexia were relatively frequent after discharge and may be considered typically related to the operation. Furthermore, we had two late intestinal occlusions caused by defects of the mesenteric folds; in both cases, surgical closure of the defect was done (one patient also had jejunal resection for intestinal necrosis). Celik et al. [13] described seven cases of diarrhea (2%) and one case of hypoglycemia. In our experience, diarrhea was rare (two cases out of 60 patients) and reactive hypoglycemia absent. The reoperation rate was between 1.3 and 7.22%, primarily caused by gallstone disease. We had two more reoperations: one abdominoplasty and one hernioplasty. The nonsurgical complication rate reported by Celik et al. was very high, with 11 patients affected by neurological complications (3.05%). However, it must be considered that all these series of SG-DD-II consisted of T2DM patients who had a long-standing clinical course and a high rate of diabetes-related complications.

12.6   Clinical Results (Table 12.1)

In our series, SG-DD-II was a highly effective bariatric surgical procedure: body weight loss was 40 ± 8 standard deviation (SD) kg at 1 year, with BMI reduction of 12 ± 4 kg/m². Percentage of excess weight loss (%EWL) was 79.3 ± 6.5%. Similar results were reported in all published experiences [13–15, 18], and SG-DD-II must be considered one of the most powerful operations available to reduce body weight in obese patients. Also, the complications of obesity are strongly affected by SG-DD-II: MS, T2DM, hypertension, and obstructive sleeping apnea syndrome resolve in the large majority of patients. If criteria for T2DM evaluation proposed by the American Diabetes Association [19] are considered, more than 90% of our patients have glycemia <100 mg/dL and glycolated hemoglobin (HbA1c) <6 % without antidiabetic medication 1 year after the operation. Similar results were reported by De Paula et al. [9, 11], Kumar et al. [10], Tinoco et al. [12], and Celik et al. [13]. Our results after 5 years, in a case-control prospective study, showed persistent T2DM remission in more than 90% of cases, with a significant difference ($p<0.01$) in comparison with the medical therapy. Only one patient was resistant to SG-DD-II, and one

Table 12.1 Clinical, biochemical, and insulin changes after DDSG-II in T2DM obese patients (reproduced with permission from [16])

Parameter	Before DDSG-II	After DDSG-II
Body weight (kg)	102.7 ± 4,2	69.5 ± 2.9**
BMI (kg/m²)	38.6 ± 2.2	26 ± 1.3**
Fasting plasma glucose (mg dL)	168.8 ± 10.3	80 ± 2.1**
HbA1c (%)	7.6 ± 0.4	5.2 ± 0.1**
Insulin (μIU/mL)	16.1 ± 3.8	2.6 ± 0.4**
Vitamin B$_{12}$ (ng/L)*	311.1 ± 33.3	332.2 ± 38.4
Folic acid (μg/L)*	6.3 ± 1.1	10.2 ± 1.8
Vitamin D (ng/mL) *	19.1 ± 2.6	15.13 ± 2.3
Total proteins (g/L)	68.1 ± 1.3	68.4 ± 0.7
Albumin (g/L)	4 0.2 ± 0.9	41.3 ± 0.7
Hemoglobin (g/dL)	13 ± 0.4	12.8 ± 0.2

DDSG-II duodenal diverted sleeve gastrectomy with ileal interposition, *T2DM* type 2 diabetes mellitus, *BMI* body mass index, *HbA1c* glycated hemoglobin
* Dietary supplementation given postoperatively
** $p<0.001$, Mann-Whitney U test

other patient relapsed 3 years after operation. Both patients had a long-lasting T2DM clinical course, with autonomic neuropathy, demonstrated by a Tilt test. We believe that T2DM patients affected by autonomic neuropathy should be excluded from this operation. Furthermore, SG-DD-II is highly effective in patients with a BMI <35 or < 30 kg/m^2 (14, 15, 17). In such patients, a large SG or fundectomy only is performed to reduce the risk of excessive weight loss, but the metabolic effects of the operation seem to be very useful for these otherwise unfavorable cases. Treatment side effects were mild; although the operation cannot be classified as malabsorptive (only a few patients had diarrhea, and none experienced protein malnutrition), since the intermediate cholesterol metabolites (like 7α-hydroxy-4-cholesten-3-one. or 7αC4) were low [16]. It is important that after SG-DD-II all patients assume a regime of daily vitamin and trace element supplementation to avoid any long-term nutritional complications.

12.7 Biochemical and Hormonal Results (Table 12.1)

After SG-DD-II, glycemic and lipidic metabolic patterns improved impressively: glycemia, low-density-lipoprotein (LDL) and total cholesterol and triglycerides decreased to normal or subnormal values [11, 20]. The restrictive effect exerted by SG and the inability of the interposed ileum to absorb lipids in the absence of the biliary salts limit caloric intake and reduce body weight. The decrease in adipose tissue induces very important changes in adipokines: leptin and resistin decrease, whereas adiponectin increases [21], restoring the best metabolic conditions to reduce lipotoxicity on the β-cell mass. Further changes induced by SG-DD-II on gastrointestinal hormones play an important role in determining the anorectic effects of the operation: the reduction of ghrelin secretion caused by SG [22] or fundectomy (in low BMI patients) and the increase in GLP-1 -2 (Fig. 12.2), PYY, and GIP [20].

These hormonal changes are also effective in regulating glucose homeostasis in T2DM patients. GLP-1 and -2, GIP, and PYY are proincretinic of insulin, whereas ghrelin is able to increase insulin resistance [23]. After SG-DD-II, fasting insulin secretion decreases and oral-glucose-stimulated insulin secretion increases (Fig. 12.3). These effects are related to the decrease of insulin resistance and the increase of β-cell sensitivity and secretion. Evaluation of β-cell function using the euglycemic hyperinsulinemic clamp with both the intravenous [24] and the oral glucose tolerance test [25] demonstrated that 1 year after the operation, SG-DD-II doubled both insulin secretion and β-cell glucose sensitivity.

SG-DD-II also changes exposure of the ileal mucosa to the biliary salts, with inhibition of 7αC4and increase of enterokine FGF-19 [19]. This hormone stimulates hepatic buildup of glycogen and reduces glucose and triglycerides in plasma, contributing to the overall metabolic effects of the operation [26].

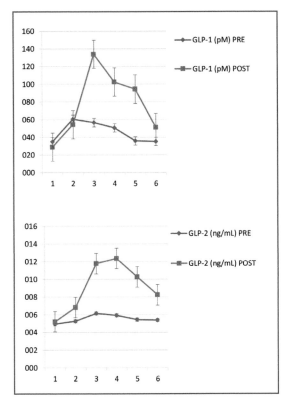

Fig. 12.2 GLP changes after SG-DD-II in obese T2DM patients. GLP-1 and GLP-2 were determined by RIA. SG-DD-II restored the ability of the enteroendocrine cells of the ileum to release GLP hormones with significant differences before and after treatment. (AUC *p*<0.01). *GLP* glucagon-like peptide, *SG-DD-II* sleeve gastrectomy-diversion of the duodenum-ileal interposition, *T2DM* type 2 diabetes mellitus, *RIA* radioimmune assay, *AUC* area under the curve

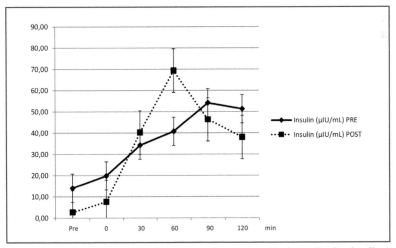

Fig. 12.3 Insulin changes after SG-DD-II in obese T2DM patients. Fasting insulin secretion is decreased after SG-DD-II as a result of reduced insulin resistance. After oral glucose load (50 g/os), insulin secretion is increased as a result of the incretinic effect of the operation (insulin was determined as RIA). The peak of insulin significantly (*p*<0.04) increased, from 40.7 ± 26 (standard deviation) to 69.2 ± 47 μIU/mL after the operation. SG-DD-II sleeve gastrectomy-diversion of the duodenum-ileal interposition, *T2DM* type 2 diabetes mellitus

12.8   Conclusions

Remission of T2DM after bariatric surgery is caused by reduction of insulin resistance and increase of insulin secretion. Weight and adipose tissue reduction is the most important factor mediating the improvement of glucose metabolism in obese patients affected by T2DM; however, the role of hormonal changes induced by surgery should also be considered. Suppression of ghrelin, the orexigenic and lipogenetic hormone secreted by the stomach fundus; stimulation of GLP-1 and -2 and PYY3-36 from endocrine enteric cells (hindgut mechanisms); and removal of foregut (still unknown) mechanisms by duodenal exclusion are recognized as very important in regulating glucose homeostasis. Ileal interposition is the most powerful operation exerting hindgut effects (incretinic stimulation) but it is unable to trigger T2DM remission. SG (which causes ghrelin suppression) in association with II seems to be a good antidiabetic operation, but the best effects occur when the duodenum is excluded from food stimulation. The technique of SG-DD-II described by De Paula et al. [3] necessitates transposition of the sleeved stomach into the submesocolic space, isoperistaltic transposition of the terminal ileum (150 cm), and restoration of the intestinal circuit by a jejunoileal anastomosis, entailing one gastric suture and three intestinal anastomoses. Operation time is long, and SG-DD-II has a complication rate higher than SG alone. However, the effects on glucose metabolism are very good, and more than 90% of patients remain in T2DM remission after 5 years of follow-up. Weight reduction is very important in obese or morbidly obese patients but is quite limited in patients with BMI <30 kg/m². For this reason, SG-DD-II should also be considered for nonobese patients affected by T2DM. Although diffusion of SG-DD-II in the clinical setting is limited, if long-term results of T2DM remission > 90% are confirmed, it would be fully considered in the surgical treatment for T2DM.

References

1. Koopmans HS, Sclafani A, Fichtner C et al (1982) The effects of ileal transposition on food intake and body weight loss in VMH-obese rats. Am J Clin Nutr 35:284–293
2. Mason EE (1999) Ileal transposition and enteroglucagon/GLP-1 in obesity (and diabetic?) surgery. Obes Surg 9:223–228
3. De Paula AL, Macedo ALV, Prudente AS et al (2006) Laparoscopic sleeve gastrectomy with ileal interposition ("neuroendocrine brake") – pilot study of a new operation. Surg Obes Relat Dis 2:464–467
4. Schubert ML (2008) Hormonal regulation of gastric acid secretion. Curr Gastroenterol Rep 10:523–527
5. Wren AM, Bloom SR (2007) Gut hormones and appetite control. Gastroenterology 132:2116–2130
6. WU T, Rayner CK, Young RL et al (2013) Gut motility and enteroendocrine secretion. Curr Opinion Pharmacol 13:928–934
7. Strader AD, Clausen TR, Goodin SZ et al (2009) Ileal interposition improves glucose tolerance in low dose streptozotocin-treated diabetic and euglycemic rats. Obes Surg 19:96–104

8. Cummings BP, Strader AD, Stanhope KL et al (2010) Ileal interposition surgery improves glucose and lipid metabolism and delays diabetes onset in the UCD-T2DM rats. Gastroenterology 138:2437–2446

9. De Paula AL, Stival AR, Halpern A et al (2011) Surgical treatment of morbid obesity: midterm outcomes of the laparoscopic ileal interposition associated to a sleeve gastrectomy in 120 patients. Obes Surg 21:668–675

10. Kumar KV, Ugale S, Gupta N et al (2011) Ileal interposition with sleeve gastrectomy for control of type 2 diabetes. Diabetes Technol Ther 11:785–789

11. De Paula AL, Stival AR, De Paula CCL et al (2010) Impact on dyslipidemia of the laparoscopic ileal interposition associated to sleeve gastrectomy in type 2 diabetic patients. J Gastrointest Surg 14:1319–1325

12. Tinoco A, El-Kadre L, Aquilar L et al (2011) Short-term and mid-term control of type 2 diabetes mellitus by laparoscopic sleeve gastrectomy with ileal interposition. World J Surg 35:238–244

13. Celik A, Ugale S, Oflouglu H et al (2015) Technical feasibility and safety profile of laparoscopic diverted sleeve gastrectomy with ileal interposition. Obes Surg 25:1184–1190

14. De Paula AL, Stival AR, Macedo A et al (2010) Prospective randomized controlled trial comparing 2 versions of laparoscopic ileal interposition associated with sleeve gastrectomy for patients with type 2 diabetes with BMI 21–34 kg/m^2. Surg Obes Relat Dis 6:296–304

15. De Paula AL, Macedo AL, Mota BR et al (2009) Laparoscopic ileal interposition associated to a diverted sleeve gastrectomy is an effective operation for the treatment of type 2 diabetes mellitus patients with BMI 21–29. Surg Endosc 23:1313–1320

16. Foschi DA, Rizzi A, Tubazio I et al (2015) Duodenal diverted sleeve gastrectomy with ileal interposition does not cause biliary salt malabsorption. Surg Obes Relat Dis 11:372–376

17. Dindo D, Demartines N, Clavien PA (2004) Classification of surgical complications. A new proposal with evaluation in a cohort of 6336 patients and results of a survey. Ann Surg 240:205–213

18. De Paula AL, Stival A, Halpern A et al (2011) Thirty-day morbidity and mortality of the laparoscopic ileal interposition associated to sleeve gastrectomy for the treatment of type 2 diabetic patients with BMI <35: an analysis of 454 consecutive patients. World J Surg 35:102–108

19. Buse JB, Caorio S, Cefalu WT et al (2009) How do we define cure of diabetes? Diabetes Care 32:2133–2135

20. De Paula AL, Macedo AL, Rassi N et al (2008) Laparoscopic treatment of metabolic syndrome in patients with type 2 diabetes mellitus. Surg Endosc 22:2670–2678

21. De Paula AL, Macedo AL, Schraibman V et al (2009) Hormonal evaluation following laparoscopic treatment of type 2 diabetes mellitus with BMI 20–34. Surg Endosc 23:1724–1732

22. Yousseif A, Emmanuel J, Karra E et al (2014) Differential effects of laparoscopic sleeve gastrectomy and laparoscopic gastric bypass on appetite, circulating acyl-ghrelin, peptide YY3-36 and active GLP-1 levels in non-diabetic humans. Obes Surg 24:241–252

23. Meek CL, Lewis HB, Reimann F et al (2016) The effect of bariatric surgery on gastrointestinal and pancreatic peptide hormones. Peptides 77:28–37

24. Vencio S, Stival A, Halpern A et al (2011) Early mechanisms of glucose improvement following laparoscopic ileal interposition associated with a sleeve gastrectomy evaluated by the euglycemic hyperinsulinemic clamp in type 2 diabetic patients with BMI below 35. Dig Surg 28:293–298

25. De Paula AL, Stival AR, Halpern A et al (2011) Improvement of insulin sensitivity and β-cell function following ileal interposition with sleeve gastrectomy in type 2 diabetic patients: potential mechanisms. J Gastroint Surg 15:1344–1353

26. Angelin B, Larsson TE, Ruddling M (2012) Circulating fibroblast growth factors as metabolic regulators. A critical appraisal. Cell Metabolism 16:693–705

The Problem of Weight Regain

13

Roberto Moroni, Marco Antonio Zappa, Giovanni Fantola,
Maria Grazia Carbonelli, and Fausta Micanti

13.1   Introduction

The effectiveness of bariatric surgery has been demonstrated, and weight loss can be simply obtained with a well-selected procedure. The real challenge of bariatric surgery success is to obtain sustained weight loss. Long-term follow-up after bariatric surgery (>5 years) is imperative to demonstrate surgical success [1]. Weight regain may occur with all three of the most common procedures (Roux-en-Y gastric bypass, sleeve gastrectomy and gastric banding), and it depends on nutritional, psychological, and surgery-related factors. There is no agreement in in the literature regarding the definition of weight regain, and it is sometimes confused with a nonspecific definition of bariatric surgery failure [2]. The percentage of excess weight loss (%EWL), percentage of weight regain, regain after the nadir reached, persistent obesity, percentage of excess body mass index loss (%EBMIL), and absolute body mass index (BMI) are definitions of renewed weight gain. A gain of %EWL <50% and an absolute BMI >35 kg/m^2 are the two most common definitions used in the literature. In order to obtain a correct diagnosis of weight regain and to treat appropriately obesity recidivism, nutritional, psychological, and surgical factors should be studied independently and in an integrated approach [3].

13.2   Homeostatic Balances in Weight Regain

Changes in energy intake, and perhaps even in energy expenditure, seen after bariatric surgery may be affected by alterations in gut and adipocyte hormones. Although it has been suggested that gut hormones such as ghrelin, glucagon-

R. Moroni (✉)
Bariatric Surgery Unit, Department of Surgery, A.O. Brotzu
Cagliari, Italy
e-mail: rob.moron@tiscali.it

L. Angrisani (Ed), Bariatric and Metabolic Surgery,
Updates in Surgery
DOI: 10.1007/ 978-88-470-3944-5_13, © Springer-Verlag Italia 2017

like peptide-1 (GLP-1), and peptide tyrosine-tyrosine (PYY) may be involved in postoperative weight homeostasis [4] due to observed decreases in ghrelin concentrations and increases in GLP-1 and PYY after Roux-en-Y gastric bypass (RYGB) and biliopancreatic diversion (BPD), other studies do not confirm a clear relationship between these changes and weight reduction [5]. A reduction in leptin and insulin serum concentrations may also play a role in weight regain [6]. Moreover, the practice of regular physical activity influence weight-loss maintenance [7]. In fact, patients who performed physical exercise on a regular basis (three or four times per week, 30-min minimum each time) show a propensity for the lowest weight regain [8]. As modifications of gastrointestinal function after surgery increase, less dietary intervention is needed to induce weight loss. In general, restrictive operations are more commonly associated with weight loss failure than are other techniques with a malabsorptive component.

From the nutritional point of view, a low glycemic load and moderately high protein content diet (or a diet based on the traditional Mediterranean dietary pattern) combined with a physical activity program has been shown to effectively treat weight regain in the short term [9]. Homeostatic eating control, regulated by macronutrients that send satiety signals to the hypothalamus, may reduce high glycemic index/low protein malnutrition, which modifies interaction between gut and hypothalamus [10]. For this reason, homeostatic eating control may play a critical role in weight regain treatment before considering redo surgery.

13.3   Nutritional Management of Weight Regain

Weight regain is most commonly related to noncompliance with dietary and lifestyle instructions (inappropriate food choices and little physical activity) both postoperatively and over the long-term follow-up [11]. Calorie intake is reduced after bariatric surgery, but it increases 1–2 years after surgery, coinciding with weight regain [12]. The problem of weight regain could be associated with dumping syndrome, a common nutritional problem after gastric bypass. Patients will often complain about lightheadedness and sweating after eating a high-glucose meal or drinking fluids during the meal. This happens because high-osmolarity foods – ice cream or pastries, for example – after bypassing much of the stomach undigested, cause an osmotic overload upon entering the small intestine. This osmotic overload brings fluid in the lumen of the small intestine, causing a vagal reaction. During this uncomfortable feeling, patients prefer to eat high-caloric-density foods to fight fatigue, thus causing insufficient weight loss or weight regain.

Nutritional and lifestyle counseling may reduce the weight of patients with previous weight regain, reducing body fat and improving the perspective of weight maintenance over time [13]. In cases of severe or unremitting postoperative weight gain, a multidisciplinary team (experienced surgeon, nutritionist, endocrinologist, psychologist, anesthetist, and specialized nurse) should consider the possibility of redo surgery.

Although bariatric surgery is not a guarantee of success, post-surgery adherence to lifestyle and nutritional recommendations – particularly to postoperative management of diet progression – and a careful nutritional follow-up could reduce the likelihood of weight regain and redo surgery in severely obese patients [14–16].

13.4   Psychologic and Psychiatric Factors of Weight Regain

There are very few studies investigating directly the clinical factors determining weight regain. All we know about the topic comes from follow-up studies that emphasize poor outcome after the first intervention, above all after banding and gastric bypass [16].

Follow-up studies at 18–24 months and 5 years after bariatric surgery [17–29] stress that the presence of a psychiatric disorder before bariatric surgery – such as panic attack [20], depression [21], personality and addiction disorder [22, 23] – can reduce weight loss and determine poor outcome, above all when these disorders were not recognized and treated at the first assessment.

Particular attention is now dedicated to the outcome of bariatric surgery for patients suffering from maladaptive eating behaviors: grazing; sweet eating; and eating disorders: binge-eating disorder (BED) and night-eating syndrome (NES) at first bariatric surgery or that develops after it.

The bariatric outcome of BED patients is still controversial. Kalarchian et al. [24] followed 96 RYGB patients for 2–7 years postsurgery and reported that in those classified as binge eaters, body mass index (BMI) increased by 5.3 kg/m^2 compared with a 2.4-kg/m^2 increase in nonbinge eaters. Impulsive behavioral traits were also a risk factor for weight regain following bariatric surgery at 2 years of follow-up [25]. On the other hand, Amianto et al. note that a BED diagnosis, once considered a major contraindication to bariatric surgery, has now been revised and that bariatric surgery interventions can now be suitable for selected BED patients treated before and after surgery, even if the extent of weight loss depends on the presence of binge episodes after the intervention [26].

Beck et al. emphasize that the weight loss obtained after bariatric surgery is less than that of nonbingers and is strictly correlated with ineffectiveness and high levels of impulsiveness that do not change in long-term follow-up studies [27]. Maladaptive eating behaviors such as grazing or sweet eating can provoke insufficient weight loss [28]. In particular, grazing is considered a high-risk behavior due to its association with medium-level impulsiveness and high anxiety levels [29]. Many studies emphasize that it can determine poor outcomes at first intervention and after bariatric surgery [30]. Often, after the first intervention, above all after sleeve gastrectomy, grazing appears as change in other eating behaviors, such as sweet, binge, or nocturnal eating. The psychopathological trait of grazing clarifies why obese patients with the disorder achieve insufficient weight loss and can also fail redo surgery without a psychiatric treatment before it. Studies on sweet-eating show that the tendency to eat sweets needs to change in the food reward system, and follow-up studies of bariatric surgery stress the low incidence of sufficient weight loss in sweet eater. Behavioral therapy before and after redo surgery seems to be effective for changing this behavior [31].

NES is characterized by a time-delayed pattern of eating relative to sleep, where most food is consumed in the evening and night. A controlled study after RYGB shows the persistence of nocturnal eating, with sufficient compliance to diet during the day [32]. Nocturnal eating (often of sweets) determines insufficient weight loss and persistence of comorbidities, such as diabetes.

Overall analysis of literature data indicates that the presence of eating disorder and maladaptive behavior determine poor outcome after the primary surgery and require a specific diagnosis and therapeutic program before redo surgery. It is essential to rule out the possibility of the patient's poor lifestyle habits being responsible for weight recidivism. Patients with binge-eating and snack-eating patterns or who consume high-caloric liquids may be at risk [33].

Bariatric surgery generally determines an improvement of psychological factors, such as cognitive impairment, body image, better relationship with others, and increased ability to cope with social pressure. However, not all patients experience a real psychological benefit after bariatric surgery. Many continue to struggle with feeling unable to comply with societal requests concerning body image. Such condition can lead to poor compliance and insufficient weight loss, thus intensifying the need for repeat surgery [34].

Redo bariatric surgery can now be considered the new challenge for surgeons, psychiatrists, psychologists, and dieticians. The reason for failure of the first intervention must be well examined, above all from a psychological perspective, and weight regain can be influenced by failure of the primary psychological assessment. Further studies are needed to highlight reasons for failure, and a more careful multidisciplinary assessment is necessary in order to initiate effective psychiatric/psychological therapies before and after redo surgery [35, 36].

13.5   Surgery-Related Factors of Weight Regain

Weight regain following bariatric surgery may be related to late complications or procedural failures. We analyzed three of the most common bariatric procedures.

13.5.1 Laparoscopic Adjustable Gastric Banding

Success with Laparoscopic adjustable gastric banding (LAGB) is closely related to appropriate follow-up, as adjustment is necessary to ensure adequate restriction and weight loss. Gastric distension with smaller quantities of food leads to an early satiation response and finally to weight loss. Since the gastric muscle is physiologically expansible, the new gastric pouch could be enlarging to accommodate food boluses. Therefore, over time, failure rates could be as high as 40–50 % [37, 38]. Patient noncompliance is the commonest cause of pouch dilatation and weight regain. In addition, surgical complications, such as slippage (8%), reduces the compressive and restrictive effects [39–41]. Premature LAGB removal is another important etiology of weight regain, as only 12% of such patients are able to maintain their reduced weight [41]. Band erosion (3.4–28%), band leak (0.6%), esophageal dilation (3.2%), port or catheter leak (7.6%), port infection (1.2%), and patient noncompliance (e.g., perhaps due to esophageal reflux) are common causes of LAGB removal [39, 42]. Some authors argue that, if successful weight loss is achieved with LAGB, band revision alone is a viable option in case of complications [39]. If the initial LAGB achieved adequate weight loss and failure was related to band slippage or pouch dilatation, laparoscopic SG (LSG) is a reasonable alternative [41]. In case of severe gastroesophageal reflux disease, band intolerance/erosion, obstruction, or insufficient weight loss, a gastric bypass or duodenal switch should be used [40, 42–44].

13.5.2 Laparoscopic Sleeve Gastrectomy

LSG is a straightforward procedure with high success rates in terms of diabetes resolution, comorbidity resolution, and weight loss. LSG has been considered a stand-alone procedure since 2008, and low-evidence studies report data about long-term follow-up weight regain [45–47]. Possible explanations for LSG failure include dilatation of the residual stomach, calibration of the stomach with an excessively large gastric bougie, and incomplete sectioning of the gastric fundus. Himpens et al. reported a %EWL of 77.5 and 53.3%, respectively, at 3- and 5-year follow-up, affirming that weight regain appears between the third and sixth postoperative year [45].

The relation between weight regain and dilation of the gastric tube is a matter of debate. Braghetto et al. [46] reported data on 15 LSG patients undergoing a gastric volumetric computed tomography (CT) scan on postoperative day 3 and between 24 and 36 months after surgery. No patient experienced weight regain with a mean remnant gastric volume increased from 108 to 250 ml.

In 2006, Langer et al. reported a series of 23 obese patients with upper gastrointestinal (GI) contrast studies at a mean follow-up of 20 months: weight regain occurred in three patients but only one presented a gastric dilatation [47]. While LSG is considered a restrictive procedure, a metabolic/malabsorptive procedure can be performed as redo surgery (i.e., gastric bypass or duodenal switch); resleeving can be proposed if gastric dilatation occurs [45].

13.5.3 Roux-en-Y Gastric Bypass

RYGB is the gold standard bariatric operation; however, a major concern in late follow-up is weight regain. Despite its success, approximately 10–20 % of patients undergoing RYGB experienced weight regain or failure to lose adequate weight at 5-year follow-up [48]. Weight loss depends on restriction of intake (gastric pouch) and metabolic/malabsorptive effects (gastrojejunal bypass). In this setting, anatomical abnormalities are postulated to play a significant role in weight regain [49, 50]. Loss of restriction caused by gastric pouch and/or gastrojejunostomy (stoma) dilatation has been shown to be responsible for loss of early satiety and weight regain in some patients [50]. Stomal dilatation is one of the common causes of weight regain. Indeed, similar to gastric pouch dilatation, stoma enlargement results in a great quantity of food being needed to distend the gastric pouch in order to obtain patient satiation.

Yimcharoen et al. demonstrated that an enlarged gastric pouch was found in almost one third of patients examined for weight regain [49]. Redo surgery in such cases could be performed to reduce pouch size and create a smaller stoma. Other options include injection of a sclerosant (sodium morrhuate) into the stoma to scar it down, endoscopic plication of the gastric pouch and stoma (StomaphyX and ROSE procedures), adding an adjustable or nonadjustable gastric band. Gastrogastric fistula is another RYGB complication resulting in weight regain. It occurs in 1.5 to 6% of patients [51]; weight regain could be dependent on loss of both restrictive and metabolic/malabsorptive components of RYGB. In gastrogastric fistula weight regain can occur over the long term. Food can travel through the correct direction (gastrojejunal anastomosis) or through the alternative direction (gastrogastric fistula); weight regain occurs when the alternative direction is preferred than the correct one [52].

13.6 Conclusions

Bariatric surgery is the most effective weight loss intervention. Despite its proven efficacy, weight regain is one of most considerable challenge after any bariatric procedure. The etiology of weight regain is multifactorial and not clearly defined. Nowadays, it is – and will become more so – an onerous public health issue, taking into account the increasingly obese global population and a constantly growing number of bariatric procedures around the world. According to the American Society for Metabolic and Bariatric Surgery (ASMBS), as much as 50% of patients regain 5% of body weight 2 years or more following their bariatric procedures, and on long-term follow-up, approximately 20–30% of patients regain most of the weight they lost [2, 53–55]. The causes leading to weight regain are multifactorial and include anatomic and psychosocial factors, physical inactivity, dietary habits, and endocrine/metabolic issues. Overall analysis of the literature indicates that benefits of redo surgery for weight regain and metabolic syndrome recidivism are greater than the risk of the new surgical procedure. It is recommended that revisional surgery be performed at a high-volume center by experienced bariatric surgeons after a careful multidisciplinary assessment of the patient's medical, nutritional, and psychopathological characteristics.

References

1. Nesset EM, Kendrick ML, Houghton SG et al (2007) A two-decade spectrum of revisional bariatric surgery at a tertiary referral center. Surg Obes Relat Dis 3:25–30
2. Mann JP, Jakes AD, Hayden JD, Barth JH (2015) Systematic review of definitions of failure in revisional bariatric surgery. Obes Surg 25:571–574
3. Brethauer SA, Kothari S, Sudan R et al (2014) Systematic review on reoperative bariatric surgery: American Society for Metabolic and Bariatric Surgery Revision Task Force. Surg Obes Relat Dis 10:952–972
4. le Roux CW, Welbourn R, Werling M et al (2007) Gut hormones as mediators of appetite and weight loss after Roux-en-Y gastric bypass. Ann Surg 246:780–785
5. Christou NV, Look D, McLean AP (2005) Pre- and post-prandial plasma ghrelin levels do not correlate with satiety or failure to achieve a successful outcome after Roux-en-Y gastric bypass. Obes Surg 15:1017–1023
6. Coupaye M, Bouillot J-L, Coussieu C et al (2005) One-year changes in energy expenditure and serum leptin following adjustable gastric banding in obese women. Obes Surg 15:827–833
7. Gerber P, Anderin C, Thorell A (2015) Weight loss prior to bariatric surgery: an updated review of the literature. Scand J Surg 104:33–39
8. Freire RH, Borges MC, Alvarez-Leite JI et al (2012) Food quality, physical activity, and nutritional follow-up as determinant of weight regain after Roux-en-Y gastric bypass. Nutrition 28:53–58
9. Faria SL, de Oliveira Kelly E, Lins RD, Faria OP (2010) Nutritional management of weight regain after bariatric surgery. Obes Surg 20:135–139
10. Schweitzer DH (2008) Adequate nutrition followed by revisional bariatric surgery to optimize homeostatic eating control. Obes Surg 18:216–219
11. Elrazek AEMAA, Elbanna AEM, Bilasy SE (2014) Medical management of patients after bariatric surgery: Principles and guidelines. World J Gastrointest Surg 6:220–228
12. Shah M, Simha V, Garg A (2006) Review: long-term impact of bariatric surgery on body weight, comorbidities, and nutritional status. J Clin Endocrinol Metab 91:4223–4231
13. Limbach KE, Ashton K, Merrell J, Heinberg LJ (2014) Relative contribution of modifiable versus non-modifiable factors as predictors of racial variance in Roux-en-Y gastric bypass weight loss outcomes. Obes Surg 24:1379–1385
14. Kuesters S, Grueneberger JM, Baumann T et al (2012) Revisionary bariatric surgery: indications and outcome of 100 consecutive operations at a single center. Surg Endosc 26:1718–1723
15. Park JY, Song D, Kim YJ (2014) Causes and outcomes of revisional bariatric surgery: initial experience at a single center. Ann Surg Treat Res 86:295–301
16. Rutledge T, Groesz LM, Savu M (2011) Psychiatric factors and weight loss patterns following gastric bypass surgery in a veteran population. Obes Surg 21:29–35
17. Burgmer R, Legenbauer T, Müller A et al (2014) Psychological outcome 4 years after restrictive bariatric surgery. Obes Surg 24:1670–1678
18. Legenbauer TM, de Zwaan M, Mühlhans B et al (2010) Do mental disorders and eating patterns affect long-term weight loss maintenance? Gen Hosp Psychiatry 32:132–140

19. Yen Y-C, Huang C-K, Tai C-M (2014) Psychiatric aspects of bariatric surgery. Curr Opin Psychiatry 27:374–379

20. de Zwaan M, Enderle J, Wagner S et al (2011) Anxiety and depression in bariatric surgery patients: a prospective, follow-up study using structured clinical interviews. J Affect Disord 133:61–68

21. Brunault P, Jacobi D, Miknius V et al (2012) High preoperative depression, phobic anxiety, and binge eating scores and low medium-term weight loss in sleeve gastrectomy obese patients: a preliminary cohort study. Psychosomatics 53:363–370

22. Odom J, Zalesin KC, Washington TL et al (2010) Behavioral predictors of weight regain after bariatric surgery. Obes Surg 20:349–356

23. Heinberg LJ, Ashton K, Coughlin J (2012) Alcohol and bariatric surgery: review and suggested recommendations for assessment and management. Surg Obes Relat Dis 8:357–363

24. Kalarchian MA, King WC, Devlin MJ et al (2015) Psychiatric disorders and weight change in a prospective study of bariatric surgery patients: a 3-year follow-up. Psychosom Med 78:373–381

25. Courcoulas AP, Yanovski SZ, Bonds D et al (2014) Long-term outcomes of bariatric surgery: a National Institutes of Health symposium. JAMA Surg 149:1323–1329

26. Amianto F, Ottone L, Abbate Daga G, Fassino S (2015) Binge-eating disorder diagnosis and treatment: a recap in front of DSM-5. BMC Psychiatry 15:70

27. Beck NN, Mehlsen M, Støving RK (2012) Psychological characteristics and associations with weight outcomes two years after gastric bypass surgery: Postoperative eating disorder symptoms are associated with weight loss outcomes. Eat Behav 13:394–397

28. Conceição E, Mitchell JE, Vaz AR et al (2014) The presence of maladaptive eating behaviors after bariatric surgery in a cross sectional study: importance of picking or nibbling on weight regain. Eat Behav 15:558–562

29. Colles SL, Dixon JB, O'Brien PE (2008) Grazing and loss of control related to eating: two high-risk factors following bariatric surgery. Obes 16:615–622

30. Meany G, Conceição E, Mitchell JE (2014) Binge eating, binge eating disorder and loss of control eating: effects on weight outcomes after bariatric surgery. Eur Eat Disord Rev 22:87–91

31. Sheets CS, Peat CM, Berg KC et al (2015) Post-operative psychosocial predictors of outcome in bariatric surgery. Obes Surg 25:330–345

32. Morrow J, Gluck M, Lorence M et al (2008) Night eating status and influence on body weight, body image, hunger, and cortisol pre- and post-Roux-en-Y Gastric Bypass (RYGB) surgery. Eat Weight Disord 13:e96–e99

33. Raman J, Smith E, Hay P (2013) The clinical obesity maintenance model: an integration of psychological constructs including mood, emotional regulation, disordered overeating, habitual cluster behaviours, health literacy and cognitive function. J Obes 2013:240128

34. Kubik JF, Gill RS, Laffin M, Karmali S (2013) The impact of bariatric surgery on psychological health. J Obes 2013:837989

35. Pataky Z, Carrard I, Golay A (2011) Psychological factors and weight loss in bariatric surgery. Curr Opin Gastroenterol 27:167–173

36. Belanger SB, Wechsler FS, Nademin ME, Virden TB (2010) Predicting outcome of gastric bypass surgery utilizing personality scale elevations, psychosocial factors, and diagnostic group membership. Obes Surg 20:1361–1371

37. Gagner M, Gentileschi P, de Csepel J et al (2002) Laparoscopic reoperative bariatric surgery: experience from 27 consecutive patients. Obes Surg 12:254–260

38. Himpens J, Cadière G-B, Bazi M et al (2011) Long-term outcomes of laparoscopic adjustable gastric banding. Arch Surg 146:802–807

39. Suter M, Calmes JM, Paroz A, Giusti V (2006) A 10-year experience with laparoscopic gastric banding for morbid obesity: high long-term complication and failure rates. Obes Surg 16:829–835

40. Ardestani A, Lautz DB, Tavakkolizadeh A (2011) Band revision versus Roux-en-Y gastric bypass conversion as salvage operation after laparoscopic adjustable gastric banding. Surg Obes Relat Dis 7:33–37

41. Bueter M, Thalheimer A, Wierlemann A, Fein M (2009) Reoperations after gastric banding: replacement or alternative procedures? Surg Endosc 23:334–340

42. Brolin RE, Cody RP (2008) Weight loss outcome of revisional bariatric operations varies according to the primary procedure. Ann Surg 248:227–232

43. Emous M, Apers J, Hoff C et al (2015) Conversion of failed laparoscopic adjustable gastric banding to Roux-en-Y gastric bypass is safe as a single-step procedure. Surg Endosc 29:2217–2223

44. Tran TT, Pauli E, Lyn-Sue JR et al (2013) Revisional weight loss surgery after failed laparoscopic gastric banding: an institutional experience. Surg Endosc 27:4087–4093

45. Himpens J, Dobbeleir J, Peeters G (2010) Long-term results of laparoscopic sleeve gastrectomy for obesity. Ann Surg 252:319–324

46. Braghetto I, Cortes C, Herquiñigo D et al (2009) Evaluation of the radiological gastric capacity and evolution of the BMI 2-3 years after sleeve gastrectomy. Obes Surg 19:1262–1269

47. Langer FB, Bohdjalian A, Felberbauer FX et al (2006) Does gastric dilatation limit the success of sleeve gastrectomy as a sole operation for morbid obesity? Obes Surg 16:166–171

48. Zingg U, McQuinn A, DiValentino D et al (2010) Revisional vs. primary Roux-en-Y gastric bypass--a case-matched analysis: less weight loss in revisions. Obes Surg 20:1627–1632

49. Yimcharoen P, Heneghan HM, Singh M et al (2011) Endoscopic findings and outcomes of revisional procedures for patients with weight recidivism after gastric bypass. Surg Endosc 25:3345–3352

50. Brethauer SA, Nfonsam V, Sherman V et al (2006) Endoscopy and upper gastrointestinal contrast studies are complementary in evaluation of weight regain after bariatric surgery. Surg Obes Relat Dis 2:643–438; discussion 649–650

51. Cucchi SG, Pories WJ, MacDonald KG, Morgan EJ (1995) Gastrogastric fistulas. A complication of divided gastric bypass surgery. Ann Surg 221:387–391

52. Filho AJB, Kondo W, Nassif LS et al (2006) Gastrogastric fistula: a possible complication of Roux-en-Y gastric bypass. JSLS 10:326–331

53. Heneghan HM, Yimcharoen P, Brethauer SA et al (2012) Influence of pouch and stoma size on weight loss after gastric bypass. Surg Obes Relat Dis 8:408–415

54. Christou NV, Look D, Maclean LD (2006) Weight gain after short- and long-limb gastric bypass in patients followed for longer than 10 years. Ann Surg 244:734–740

55. Sjöström L, Lindroos A-K, Peltonen M et al (2004) Lifestyle, diabetes, and cardiovascular risk factors 10 years after bariatric surgery. N Engl J Med 351:2683–2693

Band Revision and Conversion to Other Procedures

14

Vincenzo Borrelli and Giuliano Sarro

14.1 Introduction

Laparoscopic adjustable gastric banding (LAGB) is an effective technique that guarantees satisfactory weight loss for morbidly obese patients [1]; however, there is an increasing need for reoperation due to weight-loss failure or banding complications. In case of band complications, there are different surgical options to be considered, such as band removal or repositioning or conversion to a different procedure.

Evidence shows that when the band is removed and no additional intervention is performed, there is a very high percentage of weight regain. Rebanding has often proven to be unsuccessful, and choosing this procedure is appropriate only in cases of adequate weight loss and band leakage [2, 3]. Consequently, when LAGB results in unsatisfactory weight loss and/or a complication occurs, conversion to a different bariatric intervention should be performed. Although the best surgical solution remains undetermined, laparoscopic Roux-en-Y gastric bypass (LRYGB) and laparoscopic sleeve gastrectomy (LSG) are the two more frequently adopted procedures [4–6]. Another option is conversion to mini-gastric bypass/one anastomosis gastric bypass (MGB/OAGB) and other malabsorptive procedures.

An important factor to consider is the timing of revision. Conversion from LAGB to other procedures could be performed either in a single or a two-step approach depending on the presence of certain complications (such as erosion) that can make the stomach wall more complicated to be treated further [7–9].

In order to adopt the most successful strategy and avoid perioperative complications, it is important to review patient's overall condition and comorbidities

V. Borrelli (✉)
General and Bariatric Surgery Unit, Istituto di Cura Città di Pavia, Gruppo Ospedaliero San Donato
Pavia, Italy
e-mail: vinborr@gmail.com

L. Angrisani (Ed), Bariatric and Metabolic Surgery,
Updates in Surgery
DOI: 10.1007/ 978-88-470-3944-5_14, © Springer-Verlag Italia 2017

following a tailored multidisciplinary approach (surgeon, nutritionist, endoscopist, radiologist, and psychologist).

14.2 Technique

14.2.1 Selection and Timing of the Procedure

In order to identify the more suitable procedure for each patient, different variables must be taken into account: preoperative studies, body mass index (BMI) pre- and post-LAGB, and comorbidities, as well as patient personal preference. Patients must undergo an esophagogastroduodenoscopy to identified gastroesophageal reflux, gastric ulcers or band erosion, and an upper gastrointestinal X-ray with barium swallow to evaluate band position, pouch size, and presence of esophageal dilation. Moreover, the nutritionist's clinical investigation (anthropometrics, dietary intake, weight history) and psychologist's research for eating disorders are mandatory to identify the best procedure. Biochemical parameters, including metabolic and nutritional parameters, must also be examined.

The following conditions are suggestive for LSG:
- no hiatal hernia
- no gastroesophageal reflux disease (GERD)
- no diabetes
- iron or vitamin deficiency
- history of extensive abdominal surgery
- superobese patient programmed for staged surgery
- patient's preference.

On the other hand, the following circumstances and conditions are suggestive for LRYGB:
- hiatal hernia
- GERD
- esophageal dilation
- diabetes
- slippage or gastric pouch dilatation.

The use of malabsorptive procedures must be limited to patients failing to lose weight after gastric banding (nonresponders) without band complications. For this group, preoperative supervision by a nutritionist is highly important. Patients showing evidence of infection/slipping/erosion are more suitable for a two-step procedure. LSG is commonly performed in two steps, while LRYGB is a one-stage procedure.

14.2.2 Surgical Technique

Even if all procedures are performed like primary surgery, there are some important details to be highlighted due the presence of anatomic alterations [10, 11]. To dissect the gastric adhesions, it is convenient to be assisted by the gastric band, since the device is helpful to visualize the angle of His, provides countertension, and can be used as a guide to restore the anatomy of the proximal stomach. It is essential to remove the gastrogastric plication and totally dissect the capsule, which is a reactive scar tissue that normally builds up around an implanted LAGB. The incomplete removal of this fibrous tissue could lead to surgical stapler misfiring and staple-line leaks. For this reason, it is preferable to consider the gastric wall as very thick tissue and to use an appropriate cartridge depth; furthermore, an oversewn staple line is recommended. In case of conversion to LRYGB, gastrojejunal anastomoses either hand sewn or using a linear stapler is preferred over using a circular stapler in order to reduce the risk of stricture.

14.3 Results

Analysis and comparison of results after conversion from LAGB to LRYGB or LSG is not simple due to the high variability of data available in the literature. This is mainly caused by different indications for LAGB revision (weight regain/inadequate weight loss, band complication) and dissimilar surgical strategies (one vs. two steps). Nevertheless, from the analysis of several publications, it is clear that both procedures show positive results in terms of weight loss and comorbidity improvement. For most of the cases, results of LRYGB and LSG (as revision procedures) are as positive as those obtained after primary surgeries. The efficacy of LRYGB in terms of weight loss and comorbidity improvement is higher than LSG in different studies with an average follow-up longer than 12 months. To date, few studies have reported on conversion from LAGB to a malabsorptive bariatric procedure.

14.4 Complications

A systematic review shows that LRYGB and LSG as revisional procedures after gastric banding are relatively safe, with few complications and a very low mortality rate. However, data from the majority of publications shows that overall morbidity is significantly higher in patients who undergo LRYGB or LSG after LAGB compared with those who undergo primary procedures.

Complications after conversion are similar to those following primary LSG or LRYGB: leakage, stenosis, bleeding (grade IIIa, according to the Clavien-Dindo classification). In addition, the reoperation rate is higher for LRYGB and LSG after LAGB than for primary procedures, and the complication rate after revisional LRYGB and LSG is similar. Some studies report an increased percentage of complications, especially leak, when the conversion is performed in one step.

Table 14.1 Conversion from laparoscopic adjustable gastric banding (LAGB) to laparoscopic Roux-en-Y gastric bypass (LRYGB)

Author	Number of patients	Median follow-up	Mortality rate	Overall morbidity	Main morbidity	Reoperation	%EWL after LRYGB
Worni et al. [12]	301	NA	1/301 (0.3%)	91/301 (30.2%)	NA	11/301 (3.7%)	NA
Perathoner et al. [13]	108	3.4 + 2.5 years	0	49/108 (45.3%)	NA	9/108 (8.3%)	37.7%
Emous et al [9]	257	30 months	0	NA	21/257 (8.7%)	NA	67%
Weber et al. [14]	32	12 months	0	NA	6/32 (18.7%)	NA	NA
Jennings et al. [15]	55	2 years	0	NA	NA	NA	59.4%
Hii et al. [16]	82	1 years	1/82 (1.2%)	38/82 (46.3%)	11/82 (13.4%)	NA	50%
van Wageningen et al [17]	47	5.5 years	0	NA	8/47 (17%)	NA	NA

%EWL percentage of excess weight loss, *NA* not available

Table 14.2 Conversion from laparoscopic adjustable gastric banding (LAGB) to laparoscopic sleeve gastrectomy (LSG)

Author	Number of patients	Median follow-up	Mortality rate	Overall morbidity	Main morbidity	Reoperation	%EWL after LSG
Yazbek et al. [18]	90	12 months	0	NA	14.4%	6.6%	61.3%
Acholonu et al. [19]	15	12 months	0	NA	13.3%	6.6%	NA
Foletto et al. [20]	52	20 months	1/52 (1.9%)	NA	5.7%	NA	41.6%
Jacobs et al. [21]	32	26 months	0	NA	3.1%	NA	60%
Abu-Gazala and Keidar [22]	18	14 months	0	NA	5.5%	NA	69.7%
Dapri et al. [23]	27	18.6 months	0	NA	0	NA	34.8%
Silecchia et al. [24]	76	24 months	0	17.1%	0	0	78.5%

%EWL percentage of excess weight loss, *NA* not available

14.5   Revisional Indications

The primary considerations in revisional surgery reported in the literature [9, 12–24] are shown in Tables 14.1 and 14.2.

References

1. O'Brien PE, MacDonald L, Anderson M et al (2013) Long-term outcomes after bariatric surgery: fifteen-year follow-up of adjustable gastric banding and a systematic review of the bariatric surgical literature. Ann Surg 257:87–94
2. Suter M (2001) Laparoscopic band repositioning for pouch dilatation/slippage after gastric banding: disappointing results. Obes Surg 11:507–512
3. Müller MK, Attigah N, Wildi S et al (2008) High secondary failure rate of rebanding after failed gastric banding. Surg Endosc 22:448–453
4. Gonzalez-Heredia R, Masrur M, Patton K et al (2015) Revisions after failed gastric band: sleeve gastrectomy and Roux-en-Y gastric bypass. Surg Endosc 29:2533–2537
5. Marin-Perez P, Betancourt A, Lama A et al (2014) Outcomes after laparoscopic conversion of failed adjustable gastric banding to sleeve gastrectomy or Roux-en-Y gastric bypass. BJS 101:254–260
6. Coblijn UK, Verveld CJ, van Wagensveld BA, Lagarde SM (2013) Laparoscopic Roux-en-Y gastric bypass or laparoscopic sleeve gastrectomy as revisional procedure after adjustable gastric band: a systematic review. Obes Surg 23:1899–1914
7. Stroh C, Weiner R, Wolff S et al (2015) One- versus two-step Roux-en-Y gastric bypass after gastric banding: data analysis of the German Bariatric Surgery Registry. Obes Surg 25:755–762
8. Stroh C, Benedix D, Weiner R et al (2014) Is a one-step sleeve gastrectomy indicated as a revision procedure after gastric banding? Data analysis from a quality assurance study of the surgical treatment of obesity in Germany. Obes Surg 24:9–14
9. Emous M, Apers J, Hoff C et al (2015) Conversion of failed laparoscopic adjustable gastric banding to Roux-en-Y gastric bypass is safe as a single-step procedure. Surg Endosc 29:2217–2223
10. Fronza JS, Prystowsky JB, Hungness ES et al (2010) Revisional bariatric surgery at a single institution. Am J Surg 200:651–654
11. Hii MW, Lake AC, Kenneled C, Hopkins GH (2012) Laparoscopic conversion of failed gastric banding to Roux-en-Y gastric bypass. Short-term follow-up and technical considerations. Obes Surg 22:1022–1028
12. Worni M, Østbye T, Shah A et al (2013) High risks for adverse outcomes after gastric by-pass surgery following failed gastric banding. Ann Surg 257:279–285
13. Perathoner A, Zitt M, Lanthaler M et al (2013) Long-term follow-up evaluation of revisional gastric bypass after failed adjustable gastric banding. Surg Endosc 27:4305–4312
14. Weber M, Müller MK, Michel JM et al (2003) Laparoscopic Roux-en-Y gastric bypass, but not rebanding, should be proposed as rescue procedure for patients with failed laparoscopic gastric banding. Ann Surg 238:827–834
15. Jennings NA, Boyle M, Mahawar K et al (2013) Revisional laparoscopic RYGB following failed laparoscopic adjustable gastric banding. Obes Surg 23:947–952
16. Hii MW, Lake AC, Kenfield C, Hopkins GH (2012) Laparoscopic conversion of failed gastric banding to RYGB. Short term follow-up and technical consideration. Obes Surg 22:1022–1028
17. van Wageningen B, Berends FJ, Van Ramshorst B, Janssen IF (2006) Revision of failed laparoscopic adjustable gastric banding to Roux-en-Y gastric bypass. Obes Surg 16:137–141

18. Yazbek T, Safa N, Denis R et al (2013) Laparoscopic sleeve gastrectomy (LSG)-a good bariatric option for failed laparoscopic adjustable gastric banding(LAGB): a review of 90 patients. Obes Surg 23:300–305

19. Acholonu E, McBean E, Court I et al (2009) Safety and short-term outcomes of laparoscopic sleeve gastrectomy as a revisional approach for failed laparoscopic adjustable gastric banding in the treatment of morbid obesity. Obes Surg19:1612–1616

20. Foletto M, Prevedello L, Bernante P et al (2010) Sleeve gastrectomy as revisional procedure for failed gastric banding or gastroplasty. Surg Obes Relat Dis 6:146–151

21. Jacobs M, Gomez E, Romero R et al (2011) Failed restrictive surgery: is sleeve gastrectomy a good revisional procedure? Obes Surg 21:157–160

22. Abu-Gazala S, Keidar A (2011) Conversion of failed gastric banding into four different bariatric procedures. Surg Obes Relat Dis 8:400–407

23. Dapri G, Cadière GB, Himpens J (2009) Feasibility and technique of laparoscopic conversion of adjustable gastric banding to sleeve gastrectomy. Surg Obes Relat Dis 5:72–76

24. Silecchia G, Rizzello M, De Angelis F et al (2014) Laparoscopic sleeve gastrectomy as a revisional procedure for failed laparoscopic gastric banding with a "2-step approach": a multicenter study. Surg Obes Relat Dis 10:626-631

Sleeve Revision and Conversion to Other Procedures

15

Mirto Foletto, Alice Albanese, Maria Laura Cossu, and Paolo Bernante

15.1   Introduction

Laparoscopic sleeve gastrectomy (LSG) is one of the most common bariatric procedures performed worldwide [1, 2]. A significant worldwide rise in prevalence has been reported as 0–37% in the period 2003–2013, with LSG currently being the most frequently performed procedure in the North America and Asia/ Pacific [2]. This steep increase is probably due to the common perception of LSG as a safe and easy procedure, with no need for gastrointestinal anastomosis, short operative time, and increasing evidence of successful outcomes. Other advantages in comparison with more complex bariatric procedures have been reported, such as the absence of side effects of bypass procedures (dumping syndrome, marginal ulcers, malabsorption, small-bowel obstruction, and internal hernia) and a better quality of life over gastric banding [3, 4].

LSG consists of gastric tubulization achieved by a partial resection of the stomach on an orogastric bougie that varies in size from 32 to 40 Fr. Dissection of the greater curvature is started 4 to 6 cm proximal from the pylorus to the angle of His. The resection is completed using multiple applications of the linear stapler. The staple line can be reinforced with suture, fibrin glue, or buttress material in selected patients [5].

LSG was originally introduced as first step of a staged strategy for superobese and high-risk patients [6, 7]. Over the last decade LSG gained popularity among surgeons as a standalone primary or revisional bariatric procedure [8, 9] due to its technical feasibility, low morbidity and mortality rates, resolutions of metabolic comorbidities, excellent weight loss in the short- and mid-term, despite the

M. Foletto (✉)
Center for the Study and the Integrated Management of Obesity, Department of Medicine,
University Hospital of Padua
Padua, Italy
e-mail: mirto.foletto@unipd.it

L. Angrisani (Ed), Bariatric and Metabolic Surgery,
Updates in Surgery
DOI: 10.1007/ 978-88-470-3944-5_15, © Springer-Verlag Italia 2017

paucity of long-term data. The percentage of excess weight loss (%EWL) after 1 year is comparable with that of laparoscopic Roux-en-Y gastric bypass (LRYGB) and can exceed 70%. Comorbidity resolution is also comparable with LRYGB [10–16]. While LSG is becoming one of the leading bariatric procedures, there are still some quandaries regarding the complex management of leaks and some issues related to insufficient weight loss/weight regain and gastroesophageal reflux disease (GERD) in the long run.

Failure is usually multifactorial, involving poor patient adherence to prescribed lifestyle modifications, procedural failure, and operative error. Increasingly, as the prevalence of LSG increases, the need for robust options in revisional therapy after failure also becomes progressively more important, as occurred with adjustable gastric banding and vertical banded gastroplasty. To date, however, evidence on revision after failed LSG is limited in the literature, with the majority of available studies reporting on small patient cohorts with short-term follow-up. Actually, revisional rates range from 5.5% to 11% [17–19]. According to the Fifth International Consensus Summit for Sleeve Gastrectomy, conversions after failed sleeve due to weight-loss failure was 4.8 %, whereas it was 2.9 % due to reflux, with an overall revisional rate of 7.7% [20]. These outcomes are relevant not only for superobese patients for whom – after successful initial weight loss – a second step is offered to achieve further weight loss, but also for morbidly obese patients who underwent LSG as a stand-alone procedure or those suffering from post-LSG complications.

15.2   Reasons for LSG Conversion

15.2.1   Weight Regain or Insufficient Weight Loss

Weight regain or insufficient weight loss after LSG is a major concern, as described for other bariatric procedures. Unsatisfactory weight loss is commonly considered when the percentage of excess weight loss (%EWL) is <50% at 1-year follow-up. Dilation of the gastric tube is a point of debate. As discussed by Nedelcu et al. [21], studies on computed tomography (CT) volumetric scan of LSG would be needed to assess whether gastric dilation is secondary to an incomplete fundus resection. In their series of 61 patients, the authors describe 42 primary (gastric pouch) and 19 secondary (gastric tube) dilations following barium swallow.

Persistence of gastric fundus is not only associated with less restriction but also with persistence of high levels of ghrelin. Ghrelin is a hormone responsible of appetite during fasting, with a peak level before consumption. Ghrelin reduction is associated with less appetite and lowered calorie intake. Surgical technique is a key point to avoid incomplete fundus resection. Some tips and tricks need to be kept in mind, such as the importance of exposing the left crus of the diaphragm during the procedure, size of the orogastric bougie, and complete mobilization of the posterior gastric wall [22, 23].

15.2.2 Gastroesophageal Reflux Disease

It is still controversial whether LSG promotes, worsens, or improves reflux disease, as available data in literature are not conclusive [24–27]. Gastroesophageal reflux disease (GERD) is reported in 20–30% of sleeved patients in the long term, although Petersen et al. found an increase in lower esophageal sphincter pressure after surgery in 37 patients, which should have a protective effect against reflux after LSG [28]. A narrow sleeve can lead to GERD and dysphagia and be further worsened when a hiatal hernia is present. Stricture or angulation of the stomach at the incisura or incompetence of the lower esophageal sphincter can be important factors associated with reflux. Moreover, an undissected fundus is a major determinant risk factor for GERD. In these cases, resizing the sleeve in combination with hiatal hernia repair represents a valid treatment option, as reported by Parikh and Gagner [29]. Nedelcu et al. reported four patients with complete remission of GERD after a second gastric sleeving procedure [21]. LRYGB represents probably the most effective option to treat GERD after LSG. van Laarhoven et al. showed that patients converted to LRYGB for dysphagia or GERD were free of complaints at follow-up [30].

15.2.3 Late or Recurrent Leak/Stenosis

Late or recurrent leak usually requires surgical treatment. Surgical options may vary from conversion to LRYGB or to Roux-en-Y fistulojejunostomy and total gastrectomy, depending on fistula location and the condition of the stomach [31]. Obstruction/stricture at the incisura angularis can be successfully managed with pneumatic balloon dilation. If the procedure fails, LRYGB represents the most effective option, though successful stricturoplasty and seromyotomy have been described [32].

15.3 Revisional Procedures

Data available on LSG conversion or revision are mostly from small clinical series or short-term results. Resleeve gastrectomy (Re-LSG), one-anastomosis gastric bypass (OAGB), LRYGB, and biliopancreatic diversion-duodenal switch (BPD-DS) are all accepted options for conversion, although it is preferable to use a tailored approach to the individual patient. Recently, a case of laparoscopic diverted resleeve with ileal transposition was reported [33].

15.3.1 BPD-DS

Weiner et al. [26] showed that BPD-DS is more effective in achieving and maintaining weight loss than LRYGB, although the risk of complications and malnutrition sequelae is higher [34, 35]. BPD-DS is a well-established technique and part of a planned strategy in superobese patients [36, 37]. Iannelli reported that results in terms of weight loss of single-stage versus staged BPD-DS were similar, with an average %EWL of 73%, but in the staged approach, the risk of postoperative complications was lower [36]. Moreover, 65% of their patients had a satisfactory weight loss with primary LSG only.

15.3.2 LRYGB

Many studies show higher weight loss with conversion to BPD-DS than LRYGB. LRYGB plays an important role in resolving functional problems, such as GERD or dysphagia, after LSG. GERD symptoms mostly disappear after conversion to LRYGB, with resection of the cardial part of the sleeve to fashion a gastric pouch [13, 37]. When BPD-DS is performed without resizing the sleeve, it is unlikely to successfully resolve GERD/dysphagia.

15.3.3 Re-LSG

Re-LSG has a reasonable role when the gastric remnant is dilated or fails to give sufficient restriction [21, 29, 38]. It can also be effective in terms of weight loss and GERD resolution when some portion of the gastric fundus was left over during the primary sleeve procedure, although available data are from a small number of patients. Nedelcu et al. reported a series of 38 LSG patients converted to Re-LSG after a mean of 37.4 months, with a mean %EWL of 67% at 19.9 month follow-up [21]. Recently, Alsabah et al. [39] reported that outcomes of Re-LSG were comparable with conversion to LRYGB in terms of %EWL at 1 year (57% vs. 61.3%, p NS) in a retrospective analysis of 36 patients.

15.3.4 OAGB

OAGB was initially proposed as a primary bariatric procedure by Musella et al. in 1997 [40] and is gaining increasing acceptance among the surgical community as a primary treatment for morbid obesity, though initial concerns related to the omega reconstruction, biliary reflux, and a potential increased risk for cancer. Recently, long-term results were published by Chevallier et al. [41] on revisional OAGB after failed restrictive procedures, with a mean %EBMIL of 66% at 5 years. Though promising, it is worthwhile considering that the cohort was limited to 30 patients and that only four of them had primary LSG.

15.4 Conclusions

Morbid obesity is a chronic disease requiring lifelong therapy, and revisional surgery rates will probably continue to increase due to the higher number of bariatric procedures performed worldwide. As for other chronic comorbid diseases, some patients will respond well to initial therapy, whereas others will experience a partial response, and there will be a subset of nonresponders or who experience recurrent or persistent disease or complications.

Reoperative bariatric surgery is considered more challenging than primary procedures and is seemingly associated with a higher complication rate. Risk and complication rates are acceptable when procedures are performed by experienced surgeons. Revision and conversion procedures should be taken into consideration after failure of primary LSG — as with any other bariatric procedure — although literature data are limited.

It seems reasonable to resleeve if a dilated pouch is found on upper-gastrointestinal contrast series and good results reported in terms of weight loss. While LRYGB offers the most satisfactory results in case of refractory/de novo GERD symptoms, esophagitis, and narrowing of the incisura angularis [42], BPD-DS represents the most effective procedure as revision or the second step of a staged approach in terms of weight loss and comorbidity resolution. However, the risk of complications and malnutrition sequelae is higher. Few data are available on OAGB, although initial results are promising.

Currently, most decisions to pursue revisional bariatric surgery are based on the preference of individual surgeons and centers rather than on clear evidence. Ultimately, before these revisional options following LSG failure attain widespread acceptance as effective options to control weight regain, dedicated randomized controlled trials are required to compare long-term weight loss and complication rates, which are both significant factors in the surgeon's decision-making process. Such information with definitely provide results for an evidence-based tailored approach to redo surgery.

References

1. Ponce J, Nguyen NT, Hutter M et al (2015) American Society for Metabolic and Bariatric Surgery estimation of bariatric surgery procedures in the United States, 2011–2014. Surg Obes Relat Dis 11:1199–1200
2. Angrisani L, Santonicola A, Iovino P et al (2015) Bariatric surgery worldwide 2013. Obes Surg 25:1822–1832
3. Freeman RA, Overs SE, Zarshenas N et al (2014) Food tolerance and diet quality following adjustable gastric banding, sleeve gastrectomy and Roux-en-Y gastric bypass. Obes Res Clin Pract 8:e115–e200
4. Strain GW, Kolotkin RL, Dakin GF et al (2014) The effects of weight loss after bariatric surgery on health-related quality of life and depression. Nutr Diabetes 4:e132
5. Gagner M, Brown M (2015) Update on sleeve gastrectomy leak rate with the use of reinforcement. Obes Surg 26:146–150

6. Hess DS, Hess DW (1998) Biliopancreatic diversion with a duodenal switch. Obes Surg 8:267–282
7. Deitel M, Crosby RD, Gagner M (2008) The First International Consensus Summit for Sleeve Gastrectomy (SG), New York City, October 25–27, 2007. Obes Surg 18:487–496
8. Foletto M, Prevedello L, Bernante P et al (2010) Sleeve gastrectomy as revisional procedure for failed gastric banding or gastroplasty. Surg Obes Relat Dis 6:146–151
9. Bernante P, Foletto M, Busetto L et al (2006) Feasibility of laparoscopic sleeve gastrectomy as a revision procedure for prior laparoscopic gastric banding. Obes Surg 16:1327–1330
10. Albeladi B, Bourbao-Torunois C, Huten N (2013) Short- and midterm results between laparoscopic Roux-en-Y gastric bypass and laparoscopic sleeve gastrectomy for the treatment of morbid obesity. J Obes 2013:934653
11. D'Hondt M, Vanneste S, Pottel H et al (2011) Laparoscopic sleeve gastrectomy as a single-stage procedure for the treatment of morbid obesity and the resulting quality of life, resolution of comorbidities, food tolerance and 6-year weight loss. Surg Endosc 25:2498–2504
12. Karamanakos SN, Vagenas K, Kalfarentzos F (2008) Weight loss, appetite suppression, and changes in fasting and postprandial ghrelin and peptide-YY levels after Roux-en-Y gastric bypass and sleeve gastrectomy: a prospective, double blind study. Ann Surg 247:401–407
13. Peterli R, Borbély Y, Kern B et al (2013) Early results of the Swiss Multicentre Bypass or Sleeve Study (SM-BOSS): a prospective randomized trial comparing laparoscopic sleeve gastrectomy and Roux-en-Y gastric bypass. Ann Surg 258:690–694
14. Kehagias I, Karamanakos SN, Argentou M et al (2011) Randomized clinical trial of laparoscopic Roux-en-Y gastric bypass versus laparoscopic sleeve gastrectomy for the management of patients with BMI over 50 kg/m^2. Obes Surg 21:1650–1656
15. Leyba JL, Aulestia SN, Llopis SN (2011) Laparoscopic Roux-en-Y gastric bypass versus laparoscopic sleeve gastrectomy for the treatment of morbid obesity. A prospective study of 117 patients. Obes Surg 21:212–216
16. Fezzi M, Kolotkin RL, Nedelcu M et al (2011) Improvement in quality of life after laparoscopic sleeve gastrectomy. Obes Surg 21:1161–1167
17. Langer FB, Bohdjanlian A, Shakeri-Leidenmuhler S et al (2010) Conversion from sleeve gastrectomy to Roux-en-Y gastric bypass: indications and outcome. Obes Surg 20:835–840
18. Lacy A, Ibarzabal A, Pando E et al (2010) Revisional surgery after sleeve gastrectomy. Surg Laparosc Endosc Percutan Tech 20:351–356
19. van Rutte PW, Smulders JF, de Zoete JP, Nienhuijs SW (2012) Indications and short term outcomes or revisional surgery after failed or complicated sleeve gastrectomy. Obes Surg 22:1903–1908
20. Gagner M (2015) Fifth International Consensus Summit for Sleeve Gastrectomy: Is there a consensus? Bariatric Times 12(4 Suppl A):A22–A23
21. Nedelcu M, Noel P, Iannelli A, Gagner M (2015) Revised sleeve gastrectomy (re-sleeve). Surg Obes Relat Dis 11:1282–1288
22. Lin E, Gletsu N, Fugate K et al (2004) The effects of gastric surgery on systemic ghrelin levels in the morbidly obese. Arch Surg 139:780–784
23. Weiner RA, Weiner S, Pomhoff I et al (2007) Laparoscopic sleeve gastrectomy: influence of sleeve size and 120 resected gastric volume. Obes Surg 17:1297–1305
24. Melissas J, Braghetto I, Molina JC et al (2015) Gastroesophageal reflux disease and sleeve gastrectomy. Obes Surg 25:2430–2435
25. Stenard F, Iannelli A (2015) Laparoscopic sleeve gastrectomy and gastroesophageal reflux. World J Gastroenterol 21:10348–10357
26. Himpens J, Dobbeleir J, Peeters G (2010) Long-term results of laparoscopic sleeve gastrectomy for obesity. Ann Surg 252:319–324
27. Weiner RA, Theodoridou S, Weiner S (2011) Failure of laparoscopic sleeve gastrectomy: further procedure. Obesity Facts 4:42–46
28. Petersen WV, Meile T, Küper MA et al (2012) Functional importance of laparoscopic sleeve gastrectomy for the lower esophageal sphincter in patients with morbid obesity. Obes Surg 22:360–366

29. Parikh M, Gagner M (2008) Laparoscopic hiatal hernia repair and repeat sleeve gastrectomy for gastroesophageal reflux disease after duodenal switch. Surg Obes Relat Dis 4:73–75

30. van Laarhoven KJHM, Janssen IMC, Berends FJ (2015) Secondary surgery after sleeve gastrectomy: Roux-en-Y gastric bypass or biliopancreatic diversion with duodenal switch. Surg Obes Relat Dis 11:771–778

31. Brethauer SA, Kothari S, Sudan R et al (2014) Systematic review on reoperative bariatric surgery. Surg Obes Relat Dis 10:952–972

32. Dapri G, Cadière GB, Himpens J (2009) Laparoscopic seromyotomy for long stenosis after sleeve gastrectomy with or without duodenal switch. Obes Surg 19:495–409

33. Çelik A, Ugale S, Ofluoglu H (2015) Laparoscopic diverted resleeve with ileal transposition for failed laparoscopic sleeve gastrectomy: a case report. Surg Obes Relat Dis 11:e5–7

34. Sovik TT, Aasheim ET, Taha O et al (2011) Weight loss, cardiovascular risk factors, and quality of life after gastric bypass and duodenal switch: a randomized trial. Ann Inter Med 155:281–291

35. Botella Romero F, Milla Tobarra M, Alfaro Martinez JJ et al (2011) Bariatric surgery in duodenal switch procedure: weight changes and associated nutritional deficiencies. Endocrinol Nutr 58:214–218 [Article in Spanish]

36. Iannelli A, Schneck AS, Topart P et al (2013) Laparoscopic sleeve gastrectomy followed by duodenal switch in selected patients versus single-stage duodenal switch for superobesity: case-control study. Surg Obes Relat Dis 9:531–538

37. Dapri G, Cadiere GB, Himpens J (2011) Superobese and super-superobese patients: 2-step laparoscopic duodenal switch. Surg Obes Relat Dis 7:703–708

38. Dapri G, Cadiere GB, Himpens J (2011) Laparoscopic repeat sleeve gastrectomy versus duodenal switch after isolated sleeve gastrectomy for obesity. Surg Obes Relat Dis 7:38–43

39. AlSabah S, Alsharqawi N, Almulla A et al (2016) Approach to poor weight loss after laparoscopic sleeve gastrectomy: re-sleeve vs. gastric bypass. Obes Surg [Epub ahead of print] doi:10.1007/s11695-016-2119-y

40. Musella M, Milone M, Deitel M et al (2016) What a mini/one anastomosis gastric bypass (MGB/OAGB) is. Obes Surg 26:1322–1323

41. Chevallier JM, Arman GA, Guenzi M et al (2015) One thousand single anastomosis (omega loop) gastric bypasses to treat morbid obesity in a 7-year period: outcomes show few complications and good efficacy. Obes Surg 25:951–958

42. De Groot NL, Burgerhart JS, Van De Meeberg PC et al (2009) Systematic review: the effects of conservative and surgical treatment for obesity on gastro-oesophageal reflux disease. Aliment Pharmacol Ther 30:1091–1102

RYGB Revision and Conversion to Other Procedures

16

Daniele Tassinari, Rudj Mancini, Rosario Bellini, Rossana Berta, Carlo Moretto, Abdul Aziz Sawilah, and Marco Anselmino

16.1   Introduction

Obesity is a pathology that is rapidly increasing; the World Health Organization has, in fact, calculated that up to 10% of the world population is obese, with an estimated 2.3 billion people being overweight and 700 million being obese [1]. Bariatric surgery is universally recognized as the most efficient treatment for obesity and its related comorbidities. There is a continuous rise in the number of bariatric procedures performed worldwide, and it is estimated that 25% of patients who undergo bariatric surgery need another surgical procedure to improve quality of life and prevent reoccurrence of obesity [2, 3]. Although sleeve gastrectomy (SG) has become the most popular operation carried out in the USA, Canada, and Asia Pacific – and is increasing in popularity – Roux-en-Y gastric by-pass (RYGB), as described in a recent review by Angrisani et al. [4], despite a fall from 65.1% in 2003 to 45% in 2013, is still the most widely used surgical procedure in the world, with 95% of procedures carried out laparoscopically [4]. RYGB allows patients to achieve excellent results as far as weight loss and overall improvement are concerned, as well as resolution of related comorbidities, such as hypertension, dyslipidemia, sleep apnea, and type 2 diabetes mellitus (T2DM). However, despite the renowned efficiency of this surgical procedure, 15–35% of patients do not obtain the desired results [5–7]. For some of these patients, following a detailed multidisciplinary evaluation (psychiatrist, psychologist, endocrinologist, radiologist, bariatric surgeon), which analyzes the causes of RYGB failure, it may be opportune to propose corrective procedures. To this day, various therapeutic strategies have been

D. Tassinari (✉)
Bariatric and Metabolic Surgery Unit, Azienda Ospedaliera-Universitaria Pisana
Pisa, Italy
e-mail: tassinaridaniele@alice.it

L. Angrisani (Ed), Bariatric and Metabolic Surgery,
Updates in Surgery
DOI: 10.1007/ 978-88-470-3944-5_16, © Springer-Verlag Italia 2017

described, both endoscopic and surgical, some with the aim of incrementing the restrictive component of RYGB and others with the purpose of increasing malabsorption. The decision to propose another surgical operation to a patient who failed RYGB must be evaluated with care. In revision surgery, morbidity and mortality are higher with respect to primary bariatric procedures, and weight loss results are lower. The right choice of candidate, scrupulous preoperative evaluation, surgeon experience, and above all choice of the most appropriate revisional surgery, reduce risks and increase chances of success [8–10].

16.2   Cause of Unsatisfactory Weight Loss or Weight Regain After RYGB

Failure of RYGB can be characterized by insufficient weight loss after the operation or by acceptable weight loss followed by weight regain, which can sometimes increase back to preoperation weight and in some cases even higher than before the operation. The most widely used definition of unsatisfactory weight loss in the literature consists of percentage of excess weight loss (%EWL) <50% with a body max index (BMI) >35 kg/m^2 at 18 months postoperation [11]. Before initiating a therapeutic pathway with a patient whose RYGB has failed, it is essential to understand the causes of failure. It is particularly important to understand if technical errors have been made during the primary procedure, if there are anatomic causes that arose after surgery, or if the cause is due to the patient's behavior sabotaging the operation. In fact, according to Dykstra et al., causes of failure can be behavioral, psychological, and/or anatomical [12].

16.2.1   Behavioral Causes

By not following a diet and frequently consuming food with a high calorie count, such as fatty foods, sweets, and snacks, associated with a lack of physical exercise makes it difficult to reach the desired results and maintain them in the long term, even for patients whose operation was carried out successfully and did not present anatomic alterations. Patients need a strict follow-up with a dietician (four to five visits a year) associated with encouragement to keep a food diary (food records) and to control their weight regularly. By doing so, patients will be able to attain acceptable weight loss and maintain it over the long term [13]. Treating patients who do not show anatomic abnormality, such as gastrojejunostomy and/or gastric-pouch dilation, or a gastrogastric fistula, the reoperation for weight recidivism is destined to fail if the maladaptive behavioral problem is not treated.

16.2.2 Psychological Causes

Rutledge et al. demonstrated that obese patients with two or more related psychiatric pathologies who undergo RYGB have a 6.4-times greater probability of failure than patients with nonpsychiatric pathologies when it comes to losing weight or regaining weight 1 year after the operation [14]. Eating disorders – such as grazing, sweet eating, binge eating, or night eating – are frequent negative predictive factors of an individual's capacity to maintain weight loss; other disorders are depression, alcohol and drug abuse, and personality disorders [13, 15]. Psychiatric disorders and eating behavior should be investigated, diagnosed, and treated before primary bariatric surgery in order to predict failure. If diagnosed following weight regain, post-RYGB patients would be advised to undergo behavioral therapy. Leahey et al. sustain that behavioral therapy is not only fundamental for such patients but also gives them a greater chance to complete the behavioral treatment followed after rather than before RYGB [16].

16.2.3 Anatomical Causes

Anatomical causes are generally morphological alterations that lead to loss of the restrictive component of RYGB. The most important among these alterations are enlargement of the gastric pouch and gastrojejunostomy and the development of a gastrogastric fistula. Rawlins et al. and Heneghan et al. reported that enlargement of the gastric pouch and/or gastrojejunostomy was present in 70% of patients with weight recidivism following RYGB [17, 18]. A gastrogastric fistula is a rarer complication but is not to be neglected. It varies from 1.3% in patients whose stomach is divided at pouch formation [19] to 49% after nondivided pouch RYGB [20]. The presence of a gastrogastric fistula, which reduces the sense of early satiety, leads to weight regain and is also associated with symptoms of refractory gastroesophageal reflux disease (GERD) and marginal ulcers. Patients whose RYGB has failed due to anatomical causes are those who would benefit most from corrective surgery.

16.3   Preoperative Assessment

Evaluation of a patient who has experienced weight loss failure or weight regain after RYGB is very complex and requires collaboration of different medical professionals. A multidisciplinary evaluation is indispensable to understand the causes that led to RYGB failure and to guide the patient toward the most suitable therapeutic strategy. The main figures involved in the decision-making process are psychiatrist/psychologist, dietitian, endocrinologist, radiologist, endoscopist, and bariatric surgeon.

16.3.1 Psychological Evaluation

The psychological/psychiatric evaluation is fundamental. It is necessary to understand whether there are psychiatric diseases and/or eating disorders at the root of failure that stopped the patient from following dietary and lifestyle indications, which are indispensable to attaining and maintaining positive results. A psychologist also has the important task of understanding whether the patient's expectations in terms of weight loss after RYGB are realistic, if the patient is psychologically ready to face new surgery, is aware of the importance of follow-up, and is well prepared to follow it.

16.3.2 Dietary and Endocrinological Evaluation

The dietitian evaluates how the patient's dietary habits have changed after undergoing RYGB and if strategies to circumvent the limiting mechanisms of calorie introduction created by the operation have been applied. Patients with a restrictive mechanism that is still efficient (small gastric pouch and gastrojejunostomy) can sidestep RYGB by frequently eating small amounts of food and by eating and drinking contemporarily, which speed up progression of the alimentary bolus and consequently obtain rapid emptying of the gastric pouch (polyphagia, grazing). When proposing a new operation to these patients, it must be considered that an additional restriction would probably not be of great help. We believe that increasing the malabsorption quota through distalization of the RYGB (DRYGB) or reconversion to normal anatomy followed by SG with duodenal switch (DS), as a single or two-step procedure, is more appropriate for these patients. Other patients can, in time, force and beat the restrictions of RYGB dilating the gastric pouch and gastrojejunostomy, managing to progressively assume greater quantities of food (hyperphagia). In this case, an additional restriction is indicated. Procedures that could be proposed in this case are refashioning of the "anastomotic complex" (dilated pouch, enlarged gastrojejunostomy, and candy cane) by resecting it or using a plication suture and/or adding a band (adjustable or not). Furthermore, dumping syndrome, which is a powerful dissuader of sugar consumption in patients who suffer from it, is to be considered one mechanism by which RYGB leads to persistent loss of weight [21]. Some years after surgery, patients often no longer notice the dumping phenomenon, which leads some of them to consume an evergrowing quantity of sweet foods, which undermines the function of RYGB, even when the restrictive component is preserved. Patients diagnosed as sweet/sugar eaters, even after RYGB, should not undergo a new operation, as it is highly likely to result in one more failure. These patients should be guided toward appropriate dietary counseling.

Endocrinological evaluation is another fundamental component in the choice of appropriate surgery, especially in relation to comorbidity treatment that has demonstrated itself to be resistant to RYGB. If T2DM, dyslipidemia, or hypertension remain after RYGB, endocrinologists are likely to suggest operations with a greater component of malabsorption, such as DRYGB or biliopancreatic diversion with duodenal switch (BPD-DS) once they are sure that patients are well prepared to accept a strict follow-up and are motivated to diligently follow the nutritionist's advice to avoid the rise of serious nutritional deficiencies.

16.3.3 Upper Endoscopy and Upper Gastrointestinal Contrast Study

Detailed study of the upper gastrointestinal (GI) tract is of great value to understanding the causes of RYGB failure and to best program eventual reoperation. An upper endoscopy and a contrast upper GI study are indispensable. Endoscopy allows diagnosing the presence of a gastrogastric fistula, anastomotic ulcers, stoma enlargement, acid or bile reflux, and other signs of flaws and anatomical alterations [9]. A large gastric pouch/gastrojejunostomy has been found endoscopically in ~70% of patients with recurrent weight gain after RYGB [22].

A contrast upper GI study is also essential because it provides a dynamic image, helping define the anatomy as constructed in the primary operation, to estimate transit speed and relative gastric emptying, and to allow assess to pouch size and gastrojejunostomy diameter. In the literature, a large gastric pouch has been defined as a pouch >6 cm in length or 5 cm in width, and a wide gastrojejunostomy has been defined as an anastomosis with a diameter >2 cm. During such study, measurements must be obtained when the gastric pouch and gastrojejunostomy are maximally distended. As reported in a recent study by Wang et al., patients with images of a dilated pouch/ gastrojejunostomy are significantly more likely to benefit from a surgical reduction of pouch size or gastrojejunostomy width than from medical weight-loss programs (90% vs. 21%) [23]. Contrast upper GI study also aids in gastrogastric fistula diagnosis. Thus, according to Brethauer et al., we strongly believe that endoscopy and upper-GI contrast studies are essential and complementary in evaluating weight regain after bariatric surgery [24].

16.3.4 Surgical Evaluation

Preoperative surgical evaluation is a complex procedure given that the surgeon must to take into account multidisciplinary indications as well as the patient's needs. However, the effective technical feasibility of the operation based on local anatomical conditions after RYGB must be evaluated. Once the most appropriate operation for the patient has been identified, the surgeon must be able to consider the risks and benefits of a second operation. For technical or anatomical reasons, such as the presence of tenacious adhesions and acute or chronic tissue inflammation, the choice of redo procedure at times needs to be changed, even during surgery. When planning the surgical approach, instruments that provide the most information and that guide the technical decisions of the surgeon are review of operative notes from the primary bariatric operation, upper endoscopy, and contrast upper-GI study. A decision the surgeon must make is whether to use an open or a laparoscopic technique. In accordance with other experienced authors, such as Gagner et al. and Cohen et al., we believe that laparoscopy is feasible and safe in most revisional procedures involving the upper-GI tract, even if the primary operation was performed using the open technique [2, 25]. Tissue visualization is magnified and permits better identification of anatomical boundaries. It also reduces postoperative pain, wound complications, and length of hospital stay. At times, the presence of multiple adhesions can make revisions involving the small bowel more difficult. Extended adhesiolysis can lead to complications such as bowel perforation, ureteral injury, and bleeding. However, we believe that in expert hands, practically all cases can be dealt with laparoscopically. The choice of surgical technique must be evaluated by the surgeon according to each individual case and the surgeon's own skill and experience.

16.4   Surgical and Endoscopic Options After Failed RYGB

16.4.1   Banded or Fobi Ring Procedure and Pouch Resizing

RYGB is still the most frequent bariatric surgical procedure in the world, with a percentage of 45% of bariatric surgery procedures [4, 26]. However, in some cases, RYGB failure can come about due to insufficient body weight loss or weight regain over the years. Causes of weight gain can be the increase of intake volume determined by dilation of the gastric pouch, dilation of the anastomotic gastrojejunal complex, dilation of gastric pouch or presence of a gastrogastric fistula. However, changes in eating behavior – above all, hyperphagia – seem to be at the root of most weight gain after RYGB. Chin et al., in a preoperative radiological study [27] found no gastric pouch dilation in patients with weight regain, thus indicating salvage banding when a patient shows hyperphagic eating behavior. Salvage banding can be carried out by placing an adjustable gastric band or a nonadjustable silicone ring via laparoscopy at the gastric pouch level to restore restriction. This mechanism should be fixed with two nonabsorbable suturing stitches to the gastric pouch to avoid slippage; all studies show increased weight loss with this procedure after RYGB failure. Gobble et al. [28] reported

11 patients with an adjustable band had a mean %EWL of 20.8 ± 16.9% after an average of 13.2 ± 10.3 months; Bessler et al. [29], in 22 patients, reported percentages at 1, 2, 3, 4 and 5 years, respectively. of 29, 43.5, 51, 33, and 34%. It may be possible to reduce the number of operations for revisional surgery after gastric bypass by placing a band – adjustable or not – at the gastric pouch level during primary RYGB, especially with patients with a high BMI. Fobi [30] reported a %EWL of 69.8% at 10 years in patients who had a nonadjustable silicone band during primary RYGB. Placing a band around the gastric pouch in RYGB is also indicated for patients with reactive hypoglycemia, as it slows down gastric-pouch emptying, hence improving or resolving symptomatology. According to the literature, long-term complications can occur in ~18% of cases [26] and are represented mainly by device erosion or slippage and dysphagia, which all require removal.

Pouch and/or anastomotic gastrojejunal complex resizing are suggested in cases of RYGB failure related to anatomic dilation of the pouch, gastrojejunal anastomosis, and alimentary limb/candy cane documented on upper-GI series and after having excluded eating disorders, as mentioned above. Dilation of the gastric pouch can be divided into primary (wide construction during primary RYGB) or secondary (dilated over time). The gastric pouch can be considered dilated if – during an upper gastrointestinal endoscopy – it is possible to carry out an internal retroversion or if the horizontal diameter of the pouch, evaluated during upper-GI contrast, is 1.5 times the height of the vertebral body (2.5 cm). Gastric pouch dilation can also be evaluated on computed tomography (CT) scan with oral contrast and 3D reconstruction.

After adequate freeing of the gastric pouch and anastomotic gastrojejunal complex with left pillar exposition, the surgical technique involves a vertical gastrectomy using a linear stapler along a 36-Fr bougie. The procedure can be associated with simultaneous silicone-ring placement (Fig. 16.1). Remaking the gastrojejunal anastomosis is necessary in cases of marked anastomosis dilation, documented via gastrointestinal endoscopy, and in the presence of Roux limb dilation, documented during contrast upper-GI study. Anastomotic reconstruction associated with a fundectomy of the gastric remnant is essential in the presence of a gastrogastric fistula secondary to a perforating ulcer of the gastric pouch.

Iannelli et al. [31] demonstrated how pouch resizing was possible via laparoscopy in 90% of cases and that %EWL was, respectively, 75, 72.2, and 68.6% at 6, 12, and 18 months of follow-up, with a complication rate of 30%. However, Flanagan [32] proved that gastric-pouch enlargement is a gradual phenomenon present in all patients with RYGB and is not related to weight gain. O'Connor and Carlin [33] also showed how variation within 10–20 cm^3 in pouch dimensions is not related to weight gain. Furthermore, according to the literature, pouch resizing during secondary dilations attains lower weight loss and hence failure probably, for the reason that in these patients, an essential element at the root of RYGB failure is not anatomical dilation of the pouch but an underlying eating disorder. Therefore, placement of an adjustable gastric band,

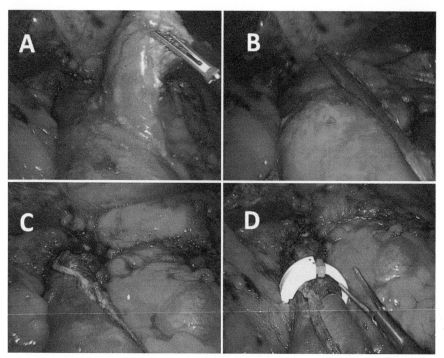

Fig. 16.1 Pouch resizing and Fobi ring placement: **A** Isolation and mobilization of the gastric pouch and anastomotic gastrojejunal complex. **B** Vertical gastrectomy using linear stapler along a 36-Fr bougie. **C** Resized gastric pouch. **D** Silicone ring placement

a nonadjustable silicone ring, or pouch resizing represents valid indications for treatment of RYGB failure. However, it is essential to select patients only after adequate psychiatric/psychological study and in relation to endoscopic procedures, X-rays, and CT with oral contrast, to be able to document dilation.

16.4.2 Endoscopic Treatment

To reduce pouch dimensions, endoscopic treatments are indicated in the presence of gastric pouch dilation or gastroenteric anastomosis as an alternative to laparoscopic or laparotomic operations. Sclerotherapy is intended increase restriction by endoscopically injecting a sclerosing substance, generally sodium morrhuate, at the perianastomotic tissue level or at gastric pouch level. Other methods, such as the Bard EndoCinch suturing system, StomaphyX, Rose, Ovesco over-the-scope clip (OTSC), and Apollo endoscopic suture system, aim to carry out a plication of the gastric wall, reducing pouch dimensions and in compliance with various fastening methods. However, there are no studies in the literature with a long-term evaluation of results of the procedures described above.

16.4.3   Conversion to Distal RYGB

An increase in the quota of malabsorption may be indicated, with the aim of optimizing weight loss, for patients who have an intact restrictive RYGB mechanism (gastric pouch volume <30 ml and gastrojejunostomy <1.5 cm) and who, during preoperative evaluation, have been diagnosed with eating disorders such as polyphagia/grazing. This can be done surgically, increasing the length of the alimentary limb, the biliopancreatic limb, or both. Distalization of the bypass consists of recreating a common limb that has a mean length of ~100–150 cm (from 75 to 300 cm depending on the author). A common channel <75 cm is not acceptable, as it carries life-threatening protein calorie malnutrition (PCM) [34]. Sugerman et al. [35] were the first to report the results of 27 conversions from RYGB to DRYGB. The alimentary limb was lengthened from 40 cm to 145 cm and, without measuring the biliopancreatic limb, anastomosed to the ileum 50–150 cm from the ileocecal valve. The first five patients had a common channel that measured 50 cm, and results in nutritional terms were catastrophic. Two patients died of hepatic failure. In the other patients, construction of a common limb of 150 cm was sufficient to avoid fatal complications. However, 18% of patients required total parenteral nutrition, and 9% eventually required a new operation to lengthen the common channel. Results in terms of weight loss were satisfactory, with a mean %EWL of 69% and complete resolution of comorbidities at 5 years after adding malabsorption. Fobi and colleagues [36] reported 65 patients who, after failed RYGB and Fobi pouch operation as first revisional procedure, were converted to DRYGB, moving the Roux limb distally halfway down the common channel (common limb: 200–300 cm). However, 23% of patients developed PCM to such an extent that it required total parenteral nutrition and/or percutaneous gastrostomy feedings, and 9% required re-revision to short-limb gastric bypass. Brolin and Cody [37] reported a series of 30 patients with unsatisfactory weight loss after RYGB and who were converted to DRYGB by detaching the biliopancreatic limb from the Roux limb, reanastomosing it to the ileum 75–100 cm proximal to the ileocecal valve, and revising or creating a new pouch/gastrojejunal anastomosis: 47.9% of patients obtained a %EWL of at least 50% at 1 year postoperatively, 7.4% developed PCM, and 3.7% had to undergo another operation to lengthen the common channel by reducing the Roux limb length to 150 cm. Rawlins et al. [17] reported a series of 29 patients who underwent conversion from a 150-cm proximal Roux limb to a DRYGB (common channel 100 cm), creating a long biliopancreatic limb. In that study, 31% of patients developed PCM, 21% required total parenteral nutrition, 27% developed nonclinical secondary hyperparathyroidism because of vitamin D deficiency, and 82 and 61% experienced vitamin D and vitamin A deficiency, respectively. One patient (3.4%) required re-revision to provide an additional 100-cm length to the common channel; mean %EWL was 68.8% at 5-year follow-up. A study recently published by Caruana et al. [38] demonstrated that conversion from RYGB to DRYGB can be carried out safely and efficiently, with an acceptable compromise between weight loss and PCM, if the percentage of bypassed intestine during revisional operation is <70%. In their study, the Roux limb was detached at the previous jejunojejunostomy, brought distally, and anastomosed to the ileum at a distance from the cecum ranging between 120 and 300 cm. A threshold of 70% of small-bowel bypassed from the food stream was identified. Patients in whom this threshold was exceeded experienced a higher percentage of PCM and diarrhea compared with those below the threshold. Patients with ≥70% of the small bowel bypassed had a mean %EWL of 47%, whereas those with <70% had a mean %EWL of 26% at 2-year follow-up. Although in terms of weight loss results were more modest, taking into account the pros and cons, exceeding the threshold of 70% is not recommended.

Revision of short-limb gastric bypass to DRYGB is a good option to enhance weight loss but is complicated by an increased incidence of PCM. We believe that the proposal by Caruana et al. [38] not to use fixed measurements when constructing the DRYGB but to personalize the operation case by case without exceeding the threshold of 70% of bypassed intestine is the safest method. However, we strongly recommend DRYGB only for selected patients who show they are able to follow the nutritional indications given and adhere to a strict follow-up program.

16.4.4 Conversion of RYGB to Biliopancreatic Diversion with Duodenal Switch

Literature shows that BPD-DS is the best operation in bariatric surgery for long-term sustained weight loss. Many studies have demonstrated that BPD-DS allows maintenance of a %EWL of 70–80%, even at 5 and 10 years from operation [39]. BPD-DS can also be suggested as revisional surgery after RYGB with the aim of optimizing weight loss by increasing the malabsorption component. This conversion should provide an additional %EWL of 15–20%, even in patients who obtained good weight loss after RYGB. Technically, conversion to BPD-DS is the most complex procedure of all possible revisions and can be done in one or two stages either open or laparoscopically. Laparoscopic conversion requires extensive experience in both advanced laparoscopy and bariatric surgery. The operation consists of two different procedures: the first one is reversing the operation back to the normal gastrointestinal anatomy followed by a sleeve gastrectomy; the second is the classic BPD-DS. The surgeon performs four anastomoses: gastrogastrostomy, duodenoileostomy, ileoileostomy, and jejunojejunostomy to reconnect the old Roux limb. It is necessary to take down the gastrojejunostomy anastomosis and to reconstruct gastric continuity with a gastrogastrostomy that can be done with a circular or linear stapler or can be hand sewn. At this point, a sleeve gastrectomy is performed along a bougie. There are differing opinions regarding appropriate bougie size [39–41]. Gagner et al. [42] suggest a 60-Fr bougie to permit adequate protein intake and digestion. Then, duodenoileostomy and ileoileostomy are performed to create a long Roux-en-Y with a 100-cm common channel and a 150-cm alimentary limb, as described by Rabkin et al. [43] or basing the Roux-en-Y construction on the percentage of total bowel length (common limb 8–12%; alimentary limb 35–45%), as suggested by Hess and Hess [44]. Finally, jejunojejunostomy of the previous RYGB is resected, and continuity is re-established by anastomosis of the biliopancreatic limb and proximal end of the old Roux limb. Given the technical complexity of the operation, even in expert hands, conversion from RYGB to BPD-DS is encumbered by a percentage of complications that cannot be neglected. Keshishian et al. [40] reported a series of 31 patients who underwent laparotomic conversion from RYGB to BPD-DS. In their study, the postoperative leak rate was 15%, and one half of the leaks required surgical intervention. Another large series of laparotomic conversions from RYGB to BPD-DS was reported by Greenbaum et al. [39]; 30% of major complications were described, including a leak rate of 22%, 2% small-bowel obstruction, 2% stenosis of the vertical sleeve, 2% duodenoenterostomy stenosis requiring endoscopic dilation, and 2% pulmonary embolism. Reoperation rate was 7%. To our knowledge, the only large series of laparoscopic conversions from RYGB to BPD-DS is the one reported by Gagner et al. [42] (12 patients). Four patients (33%) developed stricture at the gastrogastrostomy: three were performed using a circular stapler, and one was hand sewn; no leaks were reported. According to the literature, after conversion to BPD-DS, the mean %EWL at the 1- and 2-year follow-up is 59–63% and 69–77%, respectively [39, 40, 42].

We conclude that although conversion to BPD-DS for failed RYGB is highly effective, it is encumbered by a high percentage of complications that cannot be ignored. A nutritional follow-up is fundamental for these patients, together with vitamin supplements that must be taken throughout their lives, just as in primary BPD-DS.

16.5 Conclusions

RYGB is one of the most effective procedures in bariatric surgery, but treatment of failed RYGB is challenging. The first and essential step in the clinical management of these patients is to determine the reasons behind its failure. It is crucial to diagnose psychological issues, psychiatric diseases, and eating disorders that need to be treated by counseling. Equally important is to identify morphological alterations or anatomical flaws that could lead to weight regain or failure to lose weight by using upper endoscopy and contrast upper-GI study. Following an accurate preoperative evaluation, the decision to refer a patient to revisional surgery must be multidisciplinary. To this day, various surgical strategies have been described, some with the aim of adding restriction to the primary RYGB and others with the purpose of increasing malabsorption. We

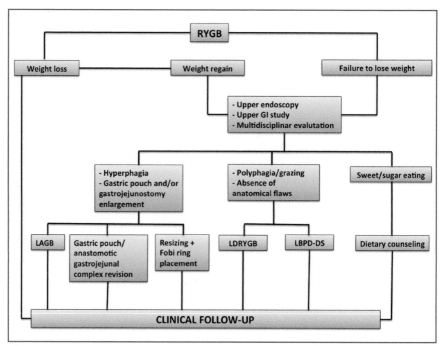

Fig. 16.2 Algorithm for treating patients with failed Roux-en-Y gastric bypass (RYGB). GI gastrointestinal, LAGB laparoscopic adjustable gastric banding, *LDRYGB* laparoscopic distal Roux-en-Y gastric bypass, *LBPD-DS* laparoscopic biliopancreatic diversion with duodenal switch

personally believe that RYGB revision and/or conversion is a safe and effective option if performed by expert surgeons in selected patients who undergo multidisciplinary assessment and who show the ability to follow nutritional indications and comply with strict follow-up program (Fig. 16.2).

References

1. Ferraz AAB, de Siqueira LT, Ferraz EM et al (2014) Revision surgery for treatment of weight regain after Roux-en-Y gastric bypass. Obes Surg 24:2–8
2. Gagner M, Gentileschi P, de Csepel J et al (2002) Laparoscopic reoperative bariatric surgery: experience from 27 consecutive patients. Obes Surg 12:254–260
3. Chousleb E, Patel S, Rosenthal R et al (2012) Reasons and operative outcomes after reversal of gastric bypass and jejunoileal bypass. Obes Surg 22:1611–1616
4. Angrisani L, Santonicola A, Scopinaro N et al (2015) Bariatric surgery worldwide 2013. Obes Surg 25:1822–1832
5. Nguyen D, Dip F, Rosenthal R et al (2015) Outcomes of revisional treatment modalities in non-complicated Roux-en-Y gastric bypass patients with weight regain. Obes Surg 25:928–934
6. Christou NV, Look D, Maclean LD (2006) Weight gain after short- and long-limb gastric bypass in patients followed for longer than 10 years. Ann Surg 244:734–740

7. Valezi AC, de Almeida Menezes M, Mali J Jr (2013) Weight loss outcome after Roux-en-Y gastric bypass: 10 years of follow-up. Obes Surg 23:1290–1293
8. Patel S, Szomstein S, Rosenthal R (2011) Reasons and outcomes of reoperative bariatric surgery for failed and complicated procedures (excluding adjustable gastric banding). Obes Surg 21:1209–1219
9. Kellogg TA (2011) Revisional bariatric surgery. Surg Clin North Am 91:1353–1371
10. Hallowell PT, Stellato TA, Yao DA et al (2009) Should bariatric revisional surgery be avoided secondary to increased morbidity and mortality? Am J Surg 197:391–396
11. Mann JP, Jakes AD, Barth JH (2015) Systematic review of definitions of failure in revisional bariatric surgery. Obes Surg 25:571–574
12. Dykstra MA, Switzer NJ, Sherman V et al (2014) Roux-en-Y gastric bypass: how and why it fails? Surgery Curr Res 4:165
13. Odom J, Zalesin KC, Hakmeh B et al (2010) Behavioral predictors of weight regain after bariatric surgery. Obes Surg 20:349–356
14. Rutledge T, Groesz LM, Savu M (2011) Psychiatric factors and weight loss patterns following gastric bypass surgery in a veteran population. Obes Surg 21:29–35
15. Livhits M, Mercado C, Dutson E et al (2012) Preoperative predictors of weight loss following bariatric surgery: systematic review. Obes Surg 22:70–89
16. Leahey TM, Bond DS, Wing RR et al (2009) When is the best time to deliver behavioral intervention to bariatric surgery patients: before or after surgery? Surg Obes Relat Dis 5:99–102
17. Rawlins ML, Teel D, Hedgcorth K, Maguire JP (2011) Revision of Roux-en-Y gastric bypass to distal bypass for failed weight loss. Surg Obes Relat Dis 7:45–49
18. Heneghan HM, Yimcharoen P, Chand B et al (2012) Influence of pouch and stoma size on weight loss after gastric bypass. Surg Obes Relat Dis 8:408–415
19. Carrodeguas L, Szomstein S, Simpfendorfer C et al (2005) Management of gastrogastric fistulas after divided Roux-en-Y gastric bypass surgery for morbid obesity: analysis of 1,292 consecutive patients and review of literature. Surg Obes Relat Dis 1:467–474
20. Capella RF, Capella JF (1999) Gastrogastric fistulas and marginal ulcers in gastric bypass procedures for weight reduction. Obes Surg 9:22–27
21. Sugerman HJ, Starkey JV, Birkenhauer R (1987) A randomized prospective trial of gastric bypass versus vertical banded gastroplasty for morbid obesity and their effects on sweets versus non-sweets eaters. Ann Surg 205:613–624
22. Yimcharoen P, Heneghan HM, Singh M et al (2011) Endoscopic findings and outcomes of revisional procedures for patients with weight recidivism after gastric bypass. Surg Endosc 25:3345–3352
23. Wang B, Levine MS, Raper S et al (2015) Utility of barium studies for patients with recurrent weight gain after Roux-en-Y gastric bypass. Clin Radiol 70:67–73
24. Brethauer SA, Nfonsam V, Sherman V et al (2006) Endoscopy and upper gastrointestinal contrast studies are complementary in evaluation of weight regain after bariatric surgery. Surg Obes Relat Dis 2:643–648
25. Cohen R, Pinheiro JS, Corres JL et al (2005) Laparoscopic revisional bariatric surgery: myths and facts. Surg Endosc 19:822–825
26. Vijgen GHEJ, Schouten R, Greve WM et al (2012) Salvage banding for failed Roux-en-Y gastric bypass. Surg Obes Relat Dis 8:803–808
27. Chin PL, Ali M, LePort PC et al (2009) Adjustable gastric band placed around gastric bypass pouch as revision operation for failed gastric bypass. Surg Obes Relat Dis 5:38–42
28. Gobble RM, Parikh MS, Fielding GA et al (2008) Gastric banding as a salvage procedure for patients with weight loss failure after Roux-en-Y gastric bypass. Surg Endosc 22:1019–1022
29. Bessler M, Daud A, DiGiorgi MF et al (2010) Adjustable gastric banding as revisional bariatric procedure after failed gastric bypass: intermediate results. Surg Obes Relat Dis 6:31–35
30. Fobi M (2005) Banded gastric bypass: combining two principles. Surg Obes Relat Dis 1:304–309

31. Iannelli A, Schneck AS, Gugenheim J et al (2013) Gastric pouch resizing for Roux-en-Y gastric bypass failure in patients with a dilated pouch. Surg Obes Relat Dis 9:260–268
32. Flanagan L (1996) Measurement of functional pouch volume following the gastric bypass procedure. Obes Surg 6:38–43
33. O'Connor EA, Carlin AM (2008) Lack of correlation between variation in small-volume gastric pouch size and weight loss after laparoscopic Roux-en-Y gastric bypass. Surg Obes Relat Dis 3:399–403
34. Brolin RE, LaMarca LB, Kenler HA et al (2002) Malabsorptive gastric bypass in patients with superobesity. J Gastrointest Surg 6:195–205
35. Sugerman HJ, Kellum JM, DeMaria EJ (1997) Conversion of proximal to distal gastric bypass for failed gastric for superobesity. J Gastrointest Surg 1:517–525
36. Fobi MA, Lee H, Igwe D et al (2001) Revision of failed gastric bypass to distal Roux-en-Y gastric bypass: a review of 65 cases. Obes Surg 11:190–195
37. Brolin RE, Cody RP (2007) Adding malabsorption for weight loss failure after gastric bypass. Surg Endosc 21:1924–1926
38. Caruana JA, Monte SV, Dandona P et al (2015) Distal small bowel bypass for weight regain after gastric bypass: safety and efficacy threshold occurs at 70% bypass. Surg Obes Relat Dis 11:1248–1256
39. Greenbaum DF, Wasser SH, Angel K et al (2011) Duodenal switch with omentopexy and feeding jejunostomy: a safe and effective revisional operation for failed previous weight loss surgery. Surg Obes Relat Dis 7:213–218
40. Keshishian A, Zahriya K, Ayagian C et al (2004) Duodenal switch is a safe operation for patients who have failed other bariatric operations. Obesity Surgery 14:1187–1192
41. Giovanni Dapri G, Cadière GB, Himpens J (2001) Laparoscopic conversion of Roux-en-Y gastric bypass to sleeve gastrectomy as first step of duodenal switch: technique and preliminary outcomes. Obes Surg 21:517–523
42. Parikh M, Pomp A, Gagner M (2007) Laparoscopic conversion of failed gastric bypass to duodenal switch: technical considerations and preliminary outcomes. Surg Obes Relat Dis 6:611–618
43. Rabkin R, Rabkin J, Becker L et al (2003) Laparoscopic technique for performing duodenal switch with gastric reduction. Obes Surg 13:263–268
44. Hess DS, Hess DW (1998) Biliopancreatic diversion with a duodenal switch. Obes Surg 8:267–282

The Problem of Gastroesophageal Reflux Disease and Hiatal Hernia

17

Paola Iovino, Antonella Santonicola, and Luigi Angrisani

17.1   Introduction

The most widely accepted definition of gastroesophageal reflux disease (GERD) is a condition that develops when stomach contents cause troublesome symptoms and/or complications [1]. GERD is a common condition with multifactorial pathogenesis affecting about 10–20% of the Western population [2]. Some contributing factors play a role in the provocation of GERD, specifically, dysfunction of the esophagogastric junction (EGJ). The EGJ consists of three components: the lower esophageal sphincter (LES), the crural diaphragm, and the anatomical flap valve. It is structurally and functionally designed to act as an antireflux barrier in which the tonically contracted smooth muscle of the LES is surrounded by oblique gastric fibers that are attached to the striated muscle of the crural diaphragm by the phrenoesophageal ligament [3]. The right crus of the diaphragm forms a sling that surrounds the distal esophagus and acts as an extrinsic sphincter by augmenting the high-pressure zone of the LES. When a proximal displacement of EGJ occurs, which is likely caused by the weakening or rupture of the phrenoesophageal ligament [4], a hiatal hernia is present because a spatial dissociation of the antireflux barrier at the EGJ into the intrinsic sphincter and extrinsic sphincter crural diaphragm exists [5]. The most comprehensive classification scheme [6] recognizes four types of hiatal hernia (Fig. 17.1):

- *Type I* or sliding hernia (>95% of cases) is characterized by a widening of the muscular hiatus and circumferential laxity of the phrenoesophageal membrane, allowing a portion of the gastric cardia to herniate upward.
- *Type II* is characterized by a localized defect in the phrenoesophageal membrane, while the gastroesophageal junction remains fixed to the preaortic fascia and the median arcuate ligament.

A. Santonicola (✉)
Gastrointestinal Unit, Department of Medicine and Surgery, University of Salerno
Salerno, Italy
e-mail: antonellasantonicola83@gmail.com

L. Angrisani (Ed), Bariatric and Metabolic Surgery,
Updates in Surgery
DOI: 10.1007/ 978-88-470-3944-5_17, © Springer-Verlag Italia 2017

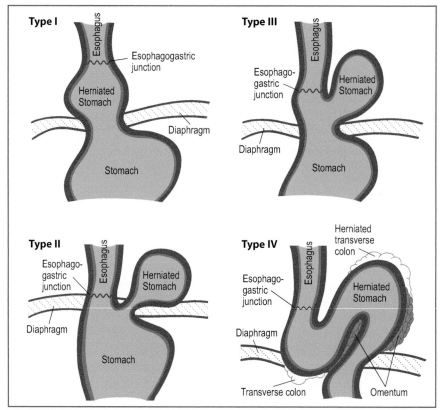

Fig. 17.1 Schematic representation of different types of hiatal hernia

- *Type III* has elements of both types I and II, with progressive enlargement of the hiatus that allows increasing amounts of fundus and LES to migrate through the hiatus.
- *Type IV* is associated with a massive defect in the phrenoesophageal membrane, allowing not only the LES and gastric fundus to herniate, but also other abdominal organs, such as the pancreas, spleen, omentum, and/or small and/or large intestine.

The presence of hiatal hernia is considered an independent risk factor for GERD [7]. It has been reported that ~75% of individuals with esophagitis and 90% of patients with Barrett's esophagus (BE) have a hiatal hernia [8, 9] Among the different types of hiatal hernia, type I (sliding) is closely associated with GERD [10]. Although sensitivity and specificity are not ideal, heartburn and regurgitation are considered typical symptoms sufficient to make a presumptive diagnosis of GERD [1], taking into account patient age and in the absence of other concerning symptoms or signs (the so-called alarm signs), which include dysphagia, odynophagia, weight loss, gastrointestinal (GI) bleeding, vomiting, family history of cancer, and epigastric mass. In such situations, upper-GI endoscopy should be considered. However, the most sensitive and objective means for assessing reflux is ambulatory 24-h pH impedance monitoring. Classically, the diagnosis of hiatal hernia relies on its presence during endoscopy or barium swallow study [11, 12]. The diagnosis of hiatal hernia with these techniques has several limitations. One limitation is that these are snapshot techniques, and the presence of a hiatal hernia is consequently considered an all-or-nothing phenomenon. Furthermore, diagnosis of a small hiatal hernia could be challenging [13]. A recent study suggests that high-resolution manometry (HRM) has a high sensitivity and specificity (92 and 93%, respectively) for detecting a hiatal hernia [13], allowing a dynamic evaluation of EGJ with a more accurate analysis. The combination of endoscopy and HRM could reach a sensitivity of 98% in the diagnosis of hiatal hernia, making it redundant to perform an additional barium esophagogram for the preoperative diagnosis of hiatal hernia. Nowadays, intraoperative findings of hiatal hernia are considered the reference standard for its diagnosis and classification [14].

17.2   GERD and Hiatal Hernia in the Obese Population

Obesity is considered an independent risk factor for GERD. Obese patients tend to have more severe erosive esophagitis and have a greater risk of developing BE and adenocarcinoma of the esophagus compared with individuals of normal weight [15, 16]. The exact pathophysiological link between obesity and GERD has not been completely determined as yet. Among the proposed mechanisms are the greater frequency of transient low esophageal sphincter relaxation (TLESR), increased prevalence of esophageal motor disorders, diminished LES pressure, as well as presence of hiatal hernia [16, 17]. Obese patients, in fact, are more than three times as likely to have hiatal hernia compared with nonobese individuals [18]. A recent study on 142 obese patients who were candidate to primary bariatric surgery [19] reveals the presence of hiatal hernia in about 23% of cases, which were, for the most part, asymptomatic. Although ~50–70% of patients undergoing bariatric surgery have asymptomatic hiatal hernia [20], obese patients show higher symptoms score, abnormal acid exposure at 24-h ambulatory pH-metry, and lower LES pressure compared with controls [21]. Other authors confirmed these data, showing that 73% of morbidly obese patients had some abnormal 24-h pH monitoring findings and 51.7% had an elevated DeMeester score [22].

In conclusion, GERD with or without hiatal hernia can manifest in a variety of forms: from no visible esophageal injury at endoscopy, also called nonerosive reflux disease (NERD), to esophageal injury or erosive reflux disease (ERD); from metaplasia of the squamous esophageal mucosa to a columnar phenotype or BE. It is not clear whether these manifestations are part of a continuous spectrum or distinct phenotypes of GERD [23, 24]. However, this wide range of clinical conditions increases the need of more preoperative investigations and influences the choice of procedure.

17.3   GERD and Bariatric Surgery

17.3.1   Gastric Banding

Literature data shows that ~80% of patients with gastric banding (GB) report resolution of GERD symptoms at short-term follow-up [25, 26]. GERD remission after GB was also evaluated using 24-h pH and manometry recordings at a mean follow-up of 19 months, revealing a significant decrease in total number of reflux episodes, total reflux time, and DeMeester score [27]. In patients with preoperative hiatal hernia, GB was performed with concomitant hiatal hernia repair with good results [28]. It has been hypothesized that the unfilled Lap-Band, when placed more proximally at the EGJ, could be an effective antireflux device, probably because it creates a longer intra-abdominal pressure zone or pulls the stomach more into the abdomen in the presence of a hiatal hernia [29]. Three years after GB, some authors described the resolution of GERD symptoms [30], whereas others reported new-onset GERD in 20.5% of patients [31]. Pouch formation is a crucial event in the occurrence of GERD after GB. Uncorrected band placement is considered the primary cause of early pouch dilation, whereas late pouch dilation is attributed to the inclusion of fundus above the band [29]. Another possible cause of GERD after GB is esophageal dilation. It is hypothesized that the inflated band reduces trans-stomal flow, causing reduced esophageal clearance, stasis of ingested food, and subsequently its reflux [32]. Given data on increased adverse outcomes, including GERD. in the long term with laparoscopic adjustable gastric banding (LAGB), as well as the high rate of reoperation or conversion to a more definitive bariatric surgery, the procedure is expected to be used less frequently going forward [33].

17.3.2   Sleeve Gastrectomy

Current data about the effect of sleeve gastrectomy (SG) on GERD are still controversial [34]. At short follow-up after SG, some authors reveal a discrete percentage of GERD remission [35, 36] and others a worsening of GERD, demonstrating a high prevalence of de novo erosive esophagitis [37] or a significant decrease of LES pressure with an increase of DeMeester score [38]. Data on long-term effects of SG are still scarce: Himpens et al [39] showed a biphasic pattern of GERD prevalence after sleeve gastrectomy, with 21.8% *de novo* proton pump inhibitor (PPI) use 1 year after SG, which improved to 3.1%

at 3 years but increased again to 23% at 6 years. In our recently study [40], we described at 5-year follow-up the resolution of GERD symptoms in 65% of patients with preoperative body mass index (BMI) ≤50 kg/m^2 and 44% in those with BMI >50 kg/m^2; we also reported new-onset GERD in 15 and 8%, respectively. Other studies reported a similar percentage of GERD resolution, from 53 to 60% [41, 42], with new-onset GERD seen in 11% of patients [41]. The reduction of weight and visceral adiposity and/or an accelerated gastric emptying might explain the positive effect of SG on GERD [34, 43]. Conversely, multiple factors may explain GERD worsening after SG [34]. One proposed mechanism is alteration of the angle of His, which normally acts as a valve to prevent reflux of stomach contents into the esophagus. Himpens et al. [39] showed that after 3 years, the rate of GERD after SG decreased, potentially due to restoration of the angle of His. Another possible factor is LES dysfunction. Specifically, after transection near the angle of His during gastrectomy, the sling fibers at the fundus are divided, which can subsequently decrease LES pressure. A significant decrease in LES pressure was, in fact, reported 3 months after SG [44]. The role of concomitant hiatal hernia repair during SG is still debated. At short term, some authors found an improvement of GERD symptoms [45, 46]. However, our recent study demonstrated no significant improvement in frequency-intensity of typical GERD symptoms in obese patients with GERD and hiatal hernia who underwent SG with concomitant hiatal hernia repair 16 ± 8 months earlier [36]. Recently, Samakar et al. [47] confirmed our results, demonstrating that at mean 2-year follow-up period, two thirds of symptomatic patients remained symptomatic after LSG with concomitant hiatal hernia repair and that 15.6 % of previously asymptomatic patients developed de novo reflux symptoms. We agree with the hypothesis of authors who suggest the routine repair of small hiatal hernias may contribute to LES dysfunction by disrupting the normal anatomical barriers to reflux in order to perform the repair. Potential repair breakdown may also lead to worsening of the hiatal hernia, given the dissection that takes place in order to perform the cruroplasty.

17.3.3 Roux-en-Y Gastric Bypass

Roux-en-Y gastric bypass (RYGB) is associated with a good outcome in regard to GERD. Symptom resolution or improvement has been described in several studies [48, 49]. Madalosso et al. [49] reported a significant reduction of GERD symptoms, reflux esophagitis, and DeMeester scores after 39 ± 7 months. The positive effect of RYGB on GERD may be explained by multiple factors. Creation of a small gastric pouch and separation of most of the stomach drastically reduce the acid that could promote regurgitation. Importantly, bile reflux is also eliminated due to biliary diversion. In fact, in patients undergoing surgery for morbid obesity, RYGB is the procedure of choice for patients with concomitant severe GERD.

A recent variation on RYGB is the omega-loop gastric bypass, also known as the mini-gastric bypass or one-anastomosis gastric bypass. There have been concerns about the proximity of the biliary flow to the gastric tube in this procedure compared with RYGB and the subsequent potential for both biliary reflux and esophagitis. However, a recent study using HRM and 24-h pH impedance monitoring performed both before and 1 year after omega-loop gastric bypass demonstrated that this procedure did not cause *de novo* gastroesophageal reflux or esophagitis [50]. Other data on the risk of developing de novo GERD after this particular procedure is needed, especially as there is a lack of studies of this procedure in obese patients with GERD.

In our opinion, in patients with a moderate to large hiatal hernia and/or severe esophagitis and/or BE, RYGB with or without hiatal hernia repair should be preferred.

References

1. Vakil N, van Zanten SV, Kahrilas P et al (2006) The Montreal definition and classification of gastroesophageal reflux disease: a global evidence-based consensus. Am J Gastroenterol 101:1900–1920
2. Katz PO, Gerson LB, Vela MF (2013) Guidelines for the diagnosis and management of gastroesophageal reflux disease. Am J Gastroenterol 108:308–328
3. van Herwaarden MA, Samsom M, Smout AJ (2004) The role of hiatus hernia in gastro-oesophageal reflux disease. Eur J Gastroenterol Hepatol 16:831–835
4. Curci JA, Melman LM, Thompson RW et al (2008) Elastic fiber depletion in the supporting ligaments of the gastroesophageal junction: a structural basis for the development of hiatal hernia. J Am Coll Surg 207:191–196
5. Sloan S, Rademaker AW, Kahrilas PJ (1992) Determinants of gastroesophageal junction incompetence: hiatal hernia, lower esophageal sphincter, or both? Ann Intern Med 117:977–982
6. Kahrilas PJ, Kim HC, Pandolfino JE (2008) Approaches to the diagnosis and grading of hiatal hernia. Best Pract Res Clin Gastroenterol 22:601–616
7. Boeckxstaens GE (2007) Review article: the pathophysiology of gastro-oesophageal reflux disease. Aliment Pharmacol Ther 26:149–160
8. Zagari RM, Fuccio L, Wallander MA et al (2008) Gastro-oesophageal reflux symptoms, oesophagitis and Barrett's oesophagus in the general population: the Loiano-Monghidoro study. Gut 57:1354–1359
9. Cameron AJ (1999) Barrett's esophagus: prevalence and size of hiatal hernia. Am J Gastroenterol 94:2054–2059
10. Hyun JJ, Bak YT (2011) Clinical significance of hiatal hernia. Gut Liver 5:267–277
11. Ott DJ, Gelfand DW, Chen YM et al (1985) Predictive relationship of hiatal hernia to reflux esophagitis. Gastrointest Radiol 10:317–320
12. Patti MG, Goldberg HI, Arcerito M et al (1996) Hiatal hernia size affects lower esophageal sphincter function, esophageal acid exposure, and the degree of mucosal injury. Am J Surg 171:182–186
13. Weijenborg PW, van Hoeij FB, Smout AJ, Bredenoord AJ (2015) Accuracy of hiatal hernia detection with esophageal high-resolution manometry. Neurogastroenterol Motil 27:293–299

14. Linke GR, Borovicka J, Schneider P et al (2008) Is a barium swallow complementary to endoscopy essential in the preoperative assessment of laparoscopic antireflux and hiatal hernia surgery? Surg Endosc 22:96–100
15. Anand G, Katz PO (2010) Gastroesophageal reflux disease and obesity. Gastroenterol Clin North Am 39:39–46
16. Hampel H, Abraham NS, El-Serag HB (2005) Meta-analysis: obesity and the risk for gastroesophageal reflux disease and its complications. Ann Intern Med 143:199–221
17. Friedenberg FK, Xanthopoulos M, Foster GD, Richter JE (2008) The association between gastroesophageal reflux disease and obesity. Am J Gastroenterol 103:2111–2122
18. Wilson LJ, Ma W, Hirschowitz BI (1999) Association of obesity with hiatal hernia and esophagitis. Am J Gastroenterol 94:2840–2844
19. Carabotti M, Avallone M, Cereatti F et al (2015) Usefulness of upper gastrointestinal symptoms as a driver to prescribe gastroscopy in obese patients candidate to bariatric surgery. A prospective study. Obes Surg 26:1075–1080
20. Anand G, Katz PO (2008) Gastroesophageal reflux disease and obesity. Rev Gastroenterol Disord 8:233–239
21. Iovino P, Angrisani L, Tremolaterra F et al (2002) Abnormal esophageal acid exposure is common in morbidly obese patients and improves after a successful LAP-BAND system implantation. Surg Endosc 16:1631–1635
22. Suter M, Dorta G, Giusti V, Calmes JM (2004) Gastro-esophageal reflux and esophageal motility disorders in morbidly obese patients. Obes Surg 14:959–966
23. Fullard M, Kang JY, Neild P et al (2006) Systematic review: does gastro-oesophageal reflux disease progress? Aliment Pharmacol Ther 24:33–45
24. Fass R, Ofman JJ (2002) Gastroesophageal reflux disease: should we adopt a new conceptual framework? Am J Gastroenterol 97:1901–1909
25. Woodman G, Cywes R, Billy H et al (2012) Effect of adjustable gastric banding on changes in gastroesophageal reflux disease (GERD) and quality of life. Curr Med Res Opin 28:581–589
26. Dixon JB, O'Brien PE (1999) Gastroesophageal reflux in obesity: the effect of LAP-BAND placement. Obes Surg 9:527–531
27. Tolonen P, Victorzon M, Niemi R, Mäkelä J (2006) Does gastric banding for morbid obesity reduce or increase gastroesophageal reflux? Obes Surg 16:1469–1474
28. Angrisani L, Iovino P, Lorenzo M et al (1999) Treatment of morbid obesity and gastroesophageal reflux with hiatal hernia by LAP-BAND. Obes Surg 9:396–398
29. de Jong JR, van Ramshorst B, Timmer R et al (2004) The influence of laparoscopic adjustable gastric banding on gastroesophageal reflux. Obes Surg 14:399–406
30. Pilone V, Vitiello A, Hasani A et al (2015) Laparoscopic adjustable gastric banding outcomes in patients with gastroesophageal reflux disease or hiatal hernia. Obes Surg 25:290–294
31. Himpens J, Dapri G, Cadière GB (2006) A prospective randomized study between laparoscopic gastric banding and laparoscopic isolated sleeve gastrectomy: results after 1 and 3 years. Obes Surg 16:1450–1456
32. Gustavsson S, Westling A (2002) Laparoscopic adjustable gastric banding: complications and side effects responsible for the poor long-term outcome. Semin Laparosc Surg 9:115–124
33. Angrisani L, Santonicola A, Iovino P et al (2015) Bariatric surgery worldwide 2013. Obes Surg 25:1822–1832
34. Laffin M, Chau J, Gill RS et al (2013) Sleeve gastrectomy and gastroesophageal reflux disease. J Obes 2013:741097
35. Melissas J, Koukouraki S, Askoxylakis J et al (2007) Sleeve gastrectomy: a restrictive procedure? Obes Surg 17:57–62
36. Santonicola A, Angrisani L, Cutolo P et al (2014) The effect of laparoscopic sleeve gastrectomy with or without hiatal hernia repair on gastroesophageal reflux disease in obese patients. Surg Obes Relat Dis 10:250–255

37. Tai CM, Huang CK, Lee YC et al (2013) Increase in gastroesophageal reflux disease symptoms and erosive esophagitis 1 year after laparoscopic sleeve gastrectomy among obese adults. Surg Endosc 27:1260–1266

38. Gorodner V, Buxhoeveden R, Clemente G et al (2015) Does laparoscopic sleeve gastrectomy have any influence on gastroesophageal reflux disease? Preliminary results. Surg Endosc 29:1760–1768

39. Himpens J, Dobbeleir J, Peeters G (2010) Long-term results of laparoscopic sleeve gastrectomy for obesity. Ann Surg 252:319–324

40. Angrisani L, Santonicola A, Hasani A et al (2015) Five-year results of laparoscopic sleeve gastrectomy: effects on gastroesophageal reflux disease symptoms and co-morbidities. Surg Obes Relat Dis pii:S1550-7289(15)00855-2

41. Rawlins MP, Brown CC, Schumacher DL (2013) Sleeve gastrectomy: 5-year outcomes of a single institution. Surg Obes Relat Dis 9:21–25

42. Hirth DA, Jones EL, Rothchild KB et al (2015) Laparoscopic sleeve gastrectomy: long-term weight loss outcomes. Surg Obes Relat Dis pii: S1550-7289(15)00049-0

43. Melissas J, Leventi A, Klinaki I et al (2013) Alterations of global gastrointestinal motility after sleeve gastrectomy: a prospective study. Ann Surg 258:976–982

44. Burgerhart JS, Schotborgh CA, Schoon EJ et al (2014) Effect of sleeve gastrectomy on gastroesophageal reflux. Obes Surg 24:1436–1441

45. Soricelli E, Iossa A, Casella G et al (2013) Sleeve gastrectomy and crural repair in obese patients with gastroesophageal reflux disease and/or hiatal hernia. Surg Obes Relat Dis 9:356–361

46. Ruscio S, Abdelgawad M, Badiali D et al (2015) Simple versus reinforced cruroplasty in patients submitted to concomitant laparoscopic sleeve gastrectomy: prospective evaluation in a bariatric center of excellence. Surg Endosc [Epub ahead of print] doi:10.1007/s00464-015-4487-0

47. Samakar K, McKenzie TJ, Tavakkoli A et al (2016) The effect of laparoscopic sleeve gastrectomy with concomitant hiatal hernia repair on gastroesophageal reflux disease in the morbidly obese. Obes Surg 26:61–66

48. Mejía-Rivas MA, Herrera-López A, Hernández-Calleros J et al (2008) Gastroesophageal reflux disease in morbid obesity: the effect of Roux-en-Y gastric bypass. Obes Surg 18:1217–1224

49. Madalosso CA, Gurski RR, Callegari-Jacques SM et al (2016) The impact of gastric bypass on gastroesophageal reflux disease in morbidly obese patients. Ann Surg 263:110–116

50. Tolone S, Cristiano S, Savarino E et al (2016) Effects of omega-loop bypass on esophago-gastric junction function. Surg Obes Relat Dis 12:62–69

51. Jeur AS (2010) Review of literatures on laparoscopic prosthetic repair of giant hiatal hernia than pure anatomical repair of crura. World J Lap Surg 3:85–90

Diabetes Surgery: Current Indications and Techniques

18

Paolo Gentileschi, Stefano D'Ugo, and Francesco Rubino

18.1 Introduction

Being pathologically overweight is an epidemic problem, with increasing numbers; global obesity rates have doubled in the last two decades, reaching 500 million in 2008. The current prevalence of 7–10% in children and adolescents is predicted to double by 2025, leading to a significant increase in obesity-related diseases [1, 2]. A large number of those patients will have multiple comorbidities, which will create a drastic negative impact on society, health-care systems, and life expectancy. Nonsurgical approaches to treating obesity, including a combination of lifestyle modifications, diets, and drugs, have shown limited long-term success. This concept is particularly true for obese people with type 2 diabetes mellitus (T2DM). The estimated worldwide prevalence of T2DM among adults was 285 million in 2010, and this is projected to increase to 439 million by 2030. Managing diabetes has historically been medical, based on lifestyle interventions combined with pharmacotherapy. However, although the pharmacological armamentarium to treat T2DM has expanded considerably, few patients are able to achieve and maintain optimal glycemic targets in the long term [3, 4].

In contrast to nonsurgical treatments, bariatric surgery has been consistently shown to induce greater and more sustained weight loss; a systematic review reported an overall percentage of excess weight loss (%EWL) of >60% with bariatric surgery and ~70 with gastric bypass. Moreover, with the widespread adoption of minimally invasive laparoscopic techniques, bariatric surgery has become safer. Current mortality risk rates are in the range of 0.2–0.5%, similar to those of other commonly performed operations, such as laparoscopic cholecystectomy [5]. Long-term results are as equally encouraging. The Swedish

P. Gentileschi (✉)
Bariatric Surgery Unit, University of Rome Tor Vergata
Rome, Italy
e-mail: gentileschi.paolo@gmail.com

L. Angrisani (Ed), Bariatric and Metabolic Surgery,
Updates in Surgery
DOI: 10.1007/ 978-88-470-3944-5_18, © Springer-Verlag Italia 2017

Obese Subjects Research Program, a nonrandomized but controlled longitudinal study, documented sustained weight loss at 10, 15 and 20 years (17, 16, and 18% respectively) in operated patients compared with minimal or no results in matched controls undergoing conventional weight loss treatment [6].

Several gastrointestinal operations have been described over recent years aimed primarily at producing significant and durable weight loss in morbidly obese patients. These procedures have also been shown in multiple trials to induce remission or dramatic improvement of T2DM and other obesity-related comorbidities. While improvement of diabetes and other metabolic disorders is an expected outcome of weight loss by any means, evidence from both experimental animal studies and clinical investigations suggests that these effects are partly independent of weight loss. This knowledge provided a rational to the idea of a "diabetes surgery" specifically aimed at treating T2DM [7]. Following this new option for diabetic patients, the concept of "metabolic surgery" has rapidly emerged in the scientific community to more broadly indicate a surgical approach aimed at controlling metabolic illnesses, not just excess weight.

Efficacy and safety of bariatric surgery to treat T2DM in obese patients have been demonstrated in many papers published in recent years. The scientific community has recommended the use of bariatric surgery in patients with diabetes and body mass index (BMI) >35 kg/m^2 and as an alternative treatment option in patients with BMI 30–35 kg/m^2 inadequately controlled with optimal medical regimens [8].

18.2   Metabolic Surgery: Mechanisms of Glycemic Control

Morbidly obese individuals with T2DM undergoing bariatric surgery reach sustained weight loss and substantial improvement in glucose metabolism. In many cases, good glycemic control is maintained without insulin injections or even medications [16, 17]. The first explanation for this effect is major weight loss; indeed, surgery is a primary trigger for increased insulin sensitivity, accompanied by cellular and tissue changes at multiple levels in the metabolism of glucose. However, growing evidence indicates that the antidiabetic mechanisms of some of these operations cannot be explained by changes in caloric intake and body weight alone. In fact, rearrangement of the gastrointestinal anatomy seems to play an important role, independently of weight loss, as shown at different levels:

• Using the duodenojejunal bypass (DJB) model in rodents, excluding the proximal small intestine (duodenum and proximal jejunum) from the passage of food contributes to the resolution (or improvement) of diabetes after other diversionary procedures [Roux-en-Y gastric bypass (RYGB), biliopancreatic diversion (BPD)] independently of weight loss.

• Diabetic patients after surgery, mainly RYGB and BPD, show a rapid improvement or resolution of T2DM long before substantial weight loss occurs.

- Different bariatric procedures can achieve similar weight loss but different glucose homeostasis. For example: RYGB achieves greater improvement of glucose tolerance and beta-cell function than an equivalent magnitude of weight loss achieved by purely gastric-restrictive bariatric surgery, such as laparoscopic adjustable gastric banding (LAGB) or following calorie restrictions.

The exact molecular mechanisms underlying improved glycemic control after gastrointestinal surgery remain unclear. In spite of anatomical and functional differences between procedures, glucose homeostasis is improved after all these types of operations, probably as an expression of partial overlap in the mechanisms of action. However, given the specific physiological role of the stomach and various intestinal segments in regulating glucose homeostasis, it is also plausible that different gastrointestinal surgeries may have distinct effects and mechanisms of action.

Several studies showed the involvement of many key peptides believed to have a role in regulating insulin secretion, including incretin peptides, especially glucagon-like peptide-1 (GLP-1) and peptide tyrosine-tyrosine (PYY) [18]. These factors are produced by intestinal enteroendocrine cells in response to ingestion of carbohydrates or fats, which in turn cause the release of insulin from the pancreas and induce satiety/reduced appetite; their changes after bariatric surgery could potentially explain the effects on obesity and diabetes. The surgical trigger for these changes is not clear; recent studies suggest the importance of modifications of gastric anatomy and physiology (emptying) more than the intestinal bypass per se [19].

One antidiabetic effect of bariatric surgery is weight independent; a number of experimental investigations have postulated changes in intestinal nutrient-sensing, regulating insulin sensitivity; disruption of vagal afferent and efferent innervations; perturbations of bile acid metabolism; taste alterations; enhancement of intestinal glucose uptake in the alimentary limb after diversionary procedures; and downregulation of one or more anti-incretin factors [7, 20–23]. However, despite much research, the exact pathway to diabetes improvement remains unidentified.

18.3   Bariatric/Metabolic Surgery in Patients with Type 2 Diabetes

18.3.1   Patients with BMI >35 kg/m²

Several papers in recent years have clearly documented results of metabolic surgery on T2DM and associated comorbidities in patients with a BMI >35 kg/m². Buchwald et al. in a meta-analysis of 22,094 diabetic patients, reported an overall 77% remission rate. The mean procedure-specific resolution of T2DM was 48%

for LAGB, 68% for vertical banded gastroplasty (VBG), 84% for RYGB, and 98% for BPD. However, these results were mainly from retrospective studies with short follow-up [5].

The multicentre Swedish Obese Subjects (SOS) study, a large prospective observational study, compared bariatric surgery LAGB (n = 156), VBG (n = 451), and RYGB (n = 34) versus conservative medical management in a group of well-matched obese patients. At 2 years, 72% of patients in the surgical group achieved remission of T2DM compared with 21% in the medically treated arm. At 10 years, the relative risk (RR) of incident T2DM was three times lower and the rates of recovery from T2DM three times greater for patients who underwent surgery compared with individuals in the control group. The proportion of individuals in whom remission was sustained at 10 years declined to 36% in the surgical group and 13% in the medical group [24].

More recently, sleeve gastrectomy (SG) has gained popularity because of its low morbidity, reasonably quick operative time, no anastomosis, and its effectiveness in obtaining effective weight loss and controlling metabolic disease. A systematic review by Gill et al. of 27 studies involving 673 patients (mean follow-up of 13.1 months) reported a T2DM resolution rate of 66.2% in obese individuals and improved glycemic control in 26.9%. This result has been confirmed by many other papers, showing that SG also represents a very effective procedure both in terms of weight reduction and control of T2DM [25].

Efficacy of bariatric/metabolic surgery has been showed also in several randomized controlled trials (RCT) comparing medical versus surgical management of T2DM. The STAMPEDE (Surgical Treatment and Medications Potentially Eradicate Diabetes Efficiently) trial compared intensive medical therapy alone versus medical therapy plus RYGB or SG in 150 obese patients (BMI 27–43 kg/m^2) with uncontrolled T2DM. The proportion of patients who reached the primary end point [glycolated hemoglobin (HbA1c) of 6.0% at 1 year) was 12% in the medical group, 42% in the RYGB group, and 37% in the SG group. No patient in the RYGB group required diabetes medications, unlike patients in the SG group (although the study was not powered to demonstrate differences between surgical procedures, these findings suggest a potentially greater antidiabetic effect of RYGB). Surgery showed a better outcome also for secondary end points, including BMI, body weight, waist circumference, and the homeostasis model assessment of insulin resistance (HOMA-IR). Although the study presented promising results, follow-up was limited to 12 months, with no reports about long-term control and risk of disease relapse [26].

In the Diabetes Surgery Study (DSS) trial, 120 patients were randomized to receive intensive lifestyle and medical therapy with or without RYGB. The primary endpoint was a composite outcome including achievement of HbA1c <7.0%, low-density lipoprotein (LDL) cholesterol <100 mg/dL, and systolic blood pressure <130 mmHg. After 12 months, 28 participants [49%; 95% confidence interval (CI) 36–63%) in the gastric bypass group and 11 (19%; 95% CI 10–32%) in the lifestyle-medical management group achieved the primary end points [27].

In 2012, a randomized clinical trial by Mingrone et al. reported results at 2 years of 60 patients (BMI ≥35 kg/m^2) with T2DM of at least 5-year duration and an HbAlc level of ≥7.0% comparing conventional medical therapy to RYGB and BPD. Diabetes remission (fasting glucose level <100 mg/dL and an HbA1c level of <6.5% in the absence of pharmacological therapy) occurred in no patient in the medical therapy group versus 75% in the RYGB group and 95% in the BPD group. All patients in the surgical group were able to discontinue pharmacotherapy (oral hypoglycemic agents and insulin) within 15 days after the operation. At 2 years, surgical patients had the greatest degree of improvement in HbA1c levels [28].

Published literature data about long-term remission of T2DM after metabolic surgery are limited. The SOS study in 2014 presented results of the prospective matched-cohort study on diabetes control and micro-macrovascular diabetes complication comparing 270 controls to 343 surgical patients. Surgery was in the form of gastric banding (GB) (61), vertical banded gastroplasty (VBG) (227), or RYGB (55). For diabetes assessment, the median follow-up time was 10 years in both groups. For diabetes complications, the median follow-up time was 17.6 and 18.1 years in control and surgery groups, respectively. Diabetes remission (defined as blood glucose <110 mg/dL and no medication) at 15 years was 6.5% for control patients and 30.4% for bariatric surgery patients ($p<0.001$). With long-term follow-up, the cumulative incidence of microvascular complications was 41.8:1000 person-years for controls and 20.6:1000 person-years in the surgery group ($p<0.001$). Macrovascular complications were observed in 44.2:1000 person-years in controls and 31.7:1000 person-years for the surgical groups($p=0.001$). This long-term data, although not randomized, shows how metabolic surgery is associated with more frequent diabetes remission and fewer complications than standard medical treatments [29].

The first longer-term results from a randomized trial were published by Mingrone et al. in 2015 [30]. The authors reported data of 5-year outcome from a trial specifically designed to assess management of T2DM comparing surgery versus medical treatments. From the group of 60 patients recruited between April and October 2009, they analyzed glycemic and metabolic control, cardiovascular risk, medication use, quality of life, and long-term complications. Overall, 19 (50%) of the 38 surgical patients [seven (37%) of 19 in the gastric bypass group and 12 (63%) of 19 in the BPD group] maintained diabetes remission at 5 years compared with none of the 15 patients in the medically treated group ($p=0.0007$). Hyperglycemia relapse occurred in eight (53%) of the 15 patients who achieved 2-year remission in the gastric bypass group and seven (37%) of the 19 patients who achieved 2-year remission in the BPD group. Eight (42%) patients who underwent gastric bypass and 13 (68%) who underwent BPD had an HbA1c concentration of ≤6.5% (≤47.5 mmol/mol) with or without medication, compared with four (27%) medically treated patients ($p=0.0457$). Surgical patients lost more weight than medically treated patients, but weight changes did not predict diabetes remission or relapse after surgery. Both surgical procedures were associated with significantly lower plasma lipids, cardiovascular risk, and medication use. Five major complications of diabetes (including one fatal myocardial infarction) arose in four (27%) patients in the medical group compared with only one complication in the gastric bypass group and no complications in the BPD group [30].

These findings show that bariatric surgery is more effective than medical treatment for the long-term control of obese patients with T2DM. Compared with medical treatments, surgery results in sustained remission of diabetes in a significant number of patients and in a greater reduction of cardiovascular risk, diabetes-related complications, and medication use, including use of insulin and cardiovascular drugs.

18.3.2   Patients with BMI <35 kg/m²

Observational studies and RCTs show with growing evidence that patients with lower BMI may obtain benefits regarding T2DM and comorbidity control following metabolic surgery. A prospective study of 66 diabetic patients with BMI 30–35 kg/m² who underwent RYGB showed remission of diabetes in ~90% and T2DM improvement in ~10% after a follow-up of 6 years. This was also associated with a cessation of pharmacotherapy for T2DM in the majority of patients and reduction of medication use (and withdrawal of insulin when previously used) in the remaining [31].

An RCT by Dixon et al. in 2008 included individuals with BMI 30–35 kg/m² comparing LAGB to medical treatment. They showed at 2-year follow-up remission of T2DM in 73% in the surgical group and 13% in the conventional therapy group; moreover, insulin sensitivity and levels of triglycerides and high-density lipoprotein (HDL) cholesterol were improved after surgery [32]. Positive results were also seen in the DSS trial including less obese patients with diagnosis of T2DM and follow-up of 12 months. Surgery was associated with greater improvement in HbA1c, LDL-cholesterol, and blood pressure that with medical treatment [27].

These preliminary results highlight the possible role of metabolic surgery even in treating T2DM in patients not classified as morbidly obese. However, despite this data, to define the exact role of surgery in this setting, more RCTs and longer follow-up results are required, along with assessments of the impact of surgery on vascular complications of diabetes.

18.4   Diabetes Surgery: A New Point of View

Over the years, the term used for surgical procedures in morbidly obese patients has been primarily "bariatric surgery." The main endpoint of these procedures is reduction of body weight and BMI. However, it became clear early that benefits and mechanisms of action of bariatric surgery extend beyond weight loss: T2DM and associated comorbidities can dramatically improve after surgery. This has led to the development of a new concept of surgery, called diabetes or metabolic surgery. The primary intent of this surgical approach is to control metabolic alterations/hyperglycemia, not only to reduce weight. This influences patient selection, with important clinical care implications. A recent study demonstrated that patients treated in metabolic surgery units have a higher incidence of T2DM and comorbidities plus lower BMI than those undergoing surgery in a bariatric unit [33]. Applying the concept of diabetes/metabolic surgery parameters to evaluate outcomes of surgery need to be redefined. Success and failure of this treatment should be assessed by remission or improvement of T2DM and associated comorbidities of the metabolic syndrome, rather than simply checking weight loss. In diabetes surgery, success parameters to consider are then no longer BMI and weight but mainly HbA1c levels, C peptide, fasting glycemia, insulin levels, lipid profile, and similar indexes.

As in other fields of medicine, diabetes and metabolic surgery means integration of knowledge and multidisciplinary expertise to provide a combination of medical and surgical treatments. These have to be seen not as alternative strategies but as complementary options, with the same goal of optimizing disease control and achieving cure when possible.

References

1. World Health Organization, Global Health Observatory (GHO) data (2008) Obesity, situation and trends. http://www.who.int/gho/ncd/risk_factors/overweight/en
2. McPherson K, Marsh T, Brown M (2007) Tackling obesities: The future choices: modelling future trends in obesity and their impact on health. UK Government Foresight Programme, Government Office for Science, London. https://www.researchgate.net/publication/242459208_Tackling_Obesities_The_Future_Choices-Modelling_Future_Trends_in_Obesity_Their_Impact_on_Health
3. Atallah R, Filion KB, Wakil SM et al (2014) Long-term effects of 4 popular diets on weight loss and cardiovascular risk factors: a systematic review of randomized controlled trials. Circ Cardiovasc Qual Outcomes 7:815–827
4. Leblanc ES, O'Connor E, Whitlock EP et al (2011) Effectiveness of primary care-relevant treatments for obesity in adults: a systematic evidence review for the US Preventive Services Task Force. Ann Intern Med 155:434–447
5. Buchwald H, Avidor Y, Braunwald E et al (2004) Bariatric surgery: a systematic review and meta-analysis. JAMA 292:1724–1737
6. Sjostrom L (2013) Review of the key results from the Swedish Obese Subjects (SOS) trial: a prospective controlled intervention study of bariatric surgery. J Intern Med 273:219–234
7. Rubino F, Gagner M (2002) Potential of surgery for curing type 2 diabetes mellitus. Ann Surg 236:554–559
8. Dixon JB, Zimmet P, Alberti KG et al (2011) Bariatric surgery for diabetes: the International Diabetes Federation takes a position. J Diabetes 3:261–264

9. Patel SR, Hakim D, Mason J, Hakim N (2013) The duodenal-jejunal bypass sleeve (Endo-Barrier Gastrointestinal Liner) for weight loss and treatment of type 2 diabetes. Surg Obes Relat Dis 9:482–484

10. Cummings BP, Strader AD, Stanhope KL et al (2010) Ileal interposition surgery improves glucose and lipid metabolism and delays diabetes onset in the UCD-T2DM rat. Gastroenterology 138:2437–2446

11. Tinoco A, El-Kadre L, Aquiar L et al (2011) Short-term and mid-term control of type 2 diabetes mellitus by laparoscopic sleeve gastrectomy with ileal interposition. World J Surg 35:2238–2244

12. Sandler BJ, Rumbaut R, Swain CP et al (2015) One-year human experience with a novel endoluminal, endoscopic gastric bypass sleeve for morbid obesity. Surg Endosc 29:3298–3303

13. Shuang J, Zhang Y, Ma L et al (2015) Relief of diabetes by duodenal-jejunal bypass sleeve implantation in the high-fat diet and streptozotocin-induced diabetic rat model is associated with an increase in GLP-1 levels and the number of GLP-1-positive cells. Exp Ther Med 10:1355–1363

14. Schumann R (2011) Anaesthesia for bariatric surgery. Best Pract Res Clin Anaesthesiol 25:83–93

15. Greenstein AJ, Wahed AS, Adeniji A et al (2012) Prevalence of adverse intraoperative events during obesity surgery and their sequelae. J Am Coll Surg 215:271–277e3

16. Rubino F, Gagner M (2002) Potential of surgery for curing type 2 diabetes mellitus. Ann Surg 236:554–559

17. Moo TA, Rubino F (2008) Gastrointestinal surgery as treatment for type 2 diabetes. Curr Opin Endocrinol Diabetes Obes 15:153–158

18. Meek CL, Lewis HB, Reimann F et al (2016) The effect of bariatric surgery on gastrointestinal and pancreatic peptide hormones. Peptides 77:28–37

19. Patel RT, Shukla AP, Ahn SM et al (2014) Surgical control of obesity and diabetes: the role of intestinal vs. gastric mechanisms in the regulation of body weight and glucose homeostasis. Obesity (Silver Spring) 22:159–169

20. Rubino F, R'bibo SL, del Genio F et al (2010) Metabolic surgery: the role of the gastrointestinal tract in diabetes mellitus. Nat Rev Endocrinol 6:102–109

21. Pournaras DJ, Glicksman C, Vincent RP et al (2012) The role of bile after Roux-en-Y gastric bypass in promoting weight loss and improving glycaemic control. Endocrinology 153:3613–3619

22. Pepino MY, Bradley D, Eagon JC et al (2014) Changes in taste perception and eating behavior after bariatric surgery-induced weight loss in women. Obesity (Silver Spring) 22:E13–20

23. Gautron L, Zechner JF, Aguirre V (2013) Vagal innervation patterns following Roux-en-Y gastric bypass in the mouse. Int J Obes (Lond) 37:1603–1607

24. Sjöström L, Lindroos AK, Peltonen M et al (2004) Swedish Obese Subjects Study Scientific Group. Lifestyle, diabetes, and cardiovascular risk factors 10 years after bariatric surgery. N Engl J Med 351:2683–2693

25. Gill RS, Birch DW, Shi X et al (2010) Sleeve gastrectomy and type 2 diabetes mellitus: a systematic review. Surg Obes Relat Dis 6:707–713

26. Schauer PR, Bhatt DL, Kirwan JP et al (2014) Bariatric surgery versus intensive medical therapy for diabetes: 3-year outcomes. N Engl J Med 370:2002–2013

27. Ikramuddin S, Korner J, Lee WJ et al (2013) Roux-en-Y gastric bypass vs intensive medical management for the control of type 2 diabetes, hypertension, and hyperlipidemia: the Diabetes Surgery Study randomized clinical trial. JAMA 309:2240–2249

28. Mingrone G, Panunzi S, De Gaetano A et al (2012) Bariatric surgery versus conventional medical therapy for type 2 diabetes. N Engl J Med 366:1577–1585

29. Sjöström L, Peltonen M, Jacobson P et al (2014) Association of bariatric surgery with long-term remission of type 2 diabetes and with microvascular and macrovascular complications. JAMA 311:2297–2304

30. Mingrone G, Panunzi S, De Gaetano A (2015) Bariatric-metabolic surgery versus conventional medical treatment in obese patients with type 2 diabetes: 5-year follow-up of an open-label, single-centre, randomised controlled trial. Lancet 386:964–973

31. Cohen RV, Pinheiro JC, Schiavon CA et al (2012) Effects of gastric bypass surgery in patients with type 2 diabetes and only mild obesity. Diabetes Care 35:1420–1428

32. Dixon JB, O'Brien PE, Playfair J et al (2008) Adjustable gastric banding and conventional therapy for type 2 diabetes: a randomized controlled trial. JAMA 299:316–323

33. Rubino F, Shukla A, Pomp A et al (2014) Bariatric, metabolic, and diabetes surgery: what's in a name? Ann Surg 259:117–122

Endoluminal Procedures

19

Giovanni Domenico De Palma, Alfredo Genco,
Massimiliano Cipriano, Gaetano Luglio, and Roberta Ienca

19.1   Introduction

Obesity is a very well recognized health-care problem worldwide due to its increasing prevalence (>35% in USA) [1], to the positive correlation between body mass index (BMI) and obesity-related comorbidities and mortality, and to huge costs related to its treatment overall (up to 21% of US health expenditures) [2]. Current treatment options include lifestyle intervention, weight-loss medications, and bariatric surgery. Lifestyle interventions, including diet and exercises, have demonstrated to be only modestly effective, with 5–10% of total body weight loss at 1 year and a significant rate of weight regain later on [3, 4]. If combined with lifestyle interventions, pharmacotherapy may lead to 5–11% of total body weight loss [5], but – with the exception of orlistat – there are no data available on weight-loss maintenance beyond 2-year follow-up due to the recent approval of some of the novel drugs by the US Food and Drug Administration (FDA).

Bariatric surgery is demonstrated to be significantly effective: gastric bypass, for example, may allow a percentage of excess weight loss (%EWL) of 62–74% at 1 year, as demonstrated in a recent meta-analysis [6], and the same review reports relatively low morbidity rates after bariatric surgery (10–17%) and a low reoperation rate (6–7%). Nevertheless, even in the minimally invasive surgery era, less than 1% of severely obese patients will ask for surgery, probably due to costs related to procedures in some countries, the fear of lack of reversibility, and the reluctance of primary care physicians to refer patients to a bariatric surgeon [7]. In this scenario, endoscopic bariatric therapy (EBT) might be considered as a further clinical tool to fill in the gap among the different treatment options. EBTs have been shown superior to lifestyle interventions alone and obesity medications; moreover, the low morbidity rate, the reversibility of some

G.D. De Palma (✉)
Department of Clinical Medicine and Surgery, University of Naples Federico II
Naples, Italy
e-mail: giovanni.depalma@unina.it

L. Angrisani (Ed), Bariatric and Metabolic Surgery,
Updates in Surgery
DOI: 10.1007/ 978-88-470-3944-5_19, © Springer-Verlag Italia 2017

procedures, and the lower BMI threshold required in order to access EBTs, might be appealing to some patients and referring physicians [6, 8]. As outlined in the 2013 guidelines by the American Heart Association (AHA)/American College of Cardiology (ACC)/The Obesity Society (TOS), EBTs are appropriate for inclusion in the obesity treatment algorithm – other than for individuals with major comorbidities wo are not ideal candidates for surgery – when lifestyle changes are not sufficient alone, when ideal BMI criteria are satisfied, and as a bridge treatment to major bariatric procedures [9].

Mechanisms of weight loss of bariatric procedures are not related to mechanical restriction or malabsorption only, as initially believed, but trigger physiological alterations in gastrointestinal (GI) motility, gut neuroendocrine system, autonomic signalling, and gut microbiota, which are also related to diabetes control. Thanks to a wide variety of novel technologies, EBTs can reproduce some anatomic alterations and consequent physiological effects of major surgical procedures proven to be effective in treating severe obesity. EBTs also offers the potential advantage of reversibility, repeatability, minimal invasiveness, and, perhaps, cost savings.

19.2   Endoscopic Bariatric Therapies

EBTs can be divided into two main groups: (1) gastric, and (2) small-bowel endoscopic interventions [10].

19.2.1 Gastric Interventions

Gastric interventions aim to reduce the gastric reservoir, thus inducing an early satiety and modulating the action of gastric mechanical and chemical receptors, orexigenic hormones, and gastric emptying.

19.2.1.1 Intragastric Balloon
Intragastric balloon (IGB) treatments are certainly the best known option, and different devices are available. This approach will be described in detail in the next section.

19.2.1.2 Aspiration Therapy
Aspiration therapy is a novel approach based on the use of a specifically designed tube, the AspireAssist (A-tube) (Aspire Bariatrics Inc, King of Prussia, PA, USA), to perform a percutaneous endoscopic gastrostomy, which is then connected to the AspireAssist device, which allows aspiration of ~30% of the meal 20 min after ingestion.

19.2.1.3 Gastroplasty Techniques

Gastroplasty attempts to decrease gastric capacity not by occupying space but by altering the gastric anatomy. Endoscopic sleeve gastroplasty (ESG) aims to reduce gastric volume by placing a series of full-thickness, closely spaced sutures through the gastric wall from the prepyloric antrum to the gastroesophageal junction using an endoscopic stitching device (OverStitch; Apollo Endosurgery Inc, Austin, TX, USA); thus, stomach volume is reduced along the greater curvature, creating a sleeve effect. Good results in terms of efficacy have been reported, with a %EWL between 30 and 40% at 6 months [11, 12]. Long-term results are awaited.

19.2.2 Small-Bowel Interventions

The second group of endoscopic procedures is represented by small-bowel interventions. The proximal small bowel plays an important role in nutrient absorption, glucose homeostasis, and production of gut peptides with entero-endocrine functions, thus regulating the sense of satiety and rate of insulin production. The mechanism of action is why bypassing this tract may help in weight loss and diabetes treatment. The EndoBarrier gastrointestinal liner system (GI Dynamics Inc, Lexington, MA, USA) aims to create a functional duodenojejunal bypass using a kind of impermeable tube-shaped Teflon liner, extending from the duodenal bulb for 65 cm into the small bowel, creating a mechanical barrier and preventing absorption of pancreaticobiliary secretions, which then will mix with food more distally in the gastrointestinal tract. The sleeve is removed endoscopically 12 months after insertion. Similarly, the gastroduodenal bypass sleeve is a 120-cm-long fluoropolymer sleeve, which is placed from the gastroesophageal junction using a combined endoscopic and laparoscopic approach. The procedure should theoretically mimic the Roux-en-Y gastric bypass, as the stomach, duodenum, and proximal jejunum are all excluded from food transit.

19.2.3 Implementation

It should be noted that most of these procedures have not been implemented in routine clinical practice or approved for bariatric indications, at least in USA. Therefore, to better define the role of such techniques in clinical scenarios, a joint task force of the American Society of Gastrointestinal Endoscopy (ASGE) and the American Society for Metabolic and Bariatric Surgery, attempted to define acceptable thresholds of safety and efficacy for EBTs. The threshold for major adverse events was set to <5%, while the threshold for efficacy as primary treatment was set at %EWL of 25% 1 year after a procedure [13].

The role of EBT as a bridge therapy should also be discussed, especially in superobese patients. Endoscopic procedures might be helpful for acute weight loss before definitive bariatric surgery in order to reduce the incidence of perioperative morbidities; moreover, EBTs might represent a further tool for selecting compliant and motivated patients, thus predicting treatment success. Emerging technologies are certainly offering a wide variety of appealing and minimally invasive treatment modalities for obesity; future research will be crucial to definitively establish the role of these novel strategies and for investigating the duration of results, the physiological mechanisms of action, the efficacy in randomized models, the cost-effectiveness profile, and the development of training and credentialing programs.

19.3   Intragastric Balloon

The IGB owes its pathophysiological concept to the original observation that patients affected by an intragastric agglomeration of partially digested hairs and vegetable fibers, otherwise known as bezoar, often complained of postprandial fullness, nausea, and vomiting. The first IGB to be marketed was the Garren-Edwards Gastric Bubble, which was approved by FDA in 1985. It was a cylinder-shaped elastomeric polyurethane balloon with a hollow central channel and a self-sealing valve located at one end. The balloon was inflated with 200 to 220 cm^3 of air, resulting in a balloon of 3 inches long and 1.75 inches in diameter with the hollow central core of 0.75 inches in diameter, through which fluid and gas could pass. The device moved freely in the stomach and had to be removed after 4 months. Within the first year of marketing of the Garren Gastric Bubble, significant problems with spontaneous deflations of the device resulting in bowel obstructions, mild gastric erosions and/or ulcers, Mallory-Weiss syndrome, and esophageal tears were reported. Moreover, several randomized trials showed no added benefits compared with sham insertion when combined with a standard weight-loss programs. Therefore, in 1992, the device was voluntarily withdrawn from the market. However, it was followed by several types of IGBs, which all showed lack of safety and efficacy. In 1987, a team of experts determined that the ideal IGB should be effective, have a soft surface, be spherical in shape, have a radiopaque valve, and be filled with liquid. The BioEnterics intragastric balloon (BIB; Allergan Inc, Irvine, CA, USA) system, in accordance with those indications, comprises a soft, transparent, silicone balloon connected by a radiopaque valve to a placement catheter with a 6.5-mm external diameter, also of soft silicone. Three fundamental factors distinguished the BIB from the 1980s bubbles: the liquid content, which made it definitely more effective; the self-sealing radiopaque valve; and the spherical form and silicone structure that rendered the complication of ulcers extremely rare. The IGB has shown to be minimally invasive, being a removable device with a high safety and efficacy profile. To date the BIB – and recently its evolution, the Orbera intragastric balloon, sold by Apollo Endosurgery (Austin, TX, USA) – remains the most frequently used and best known brand, although several types of balloons (Heliosphere bag, Spatz adjustable intragastric balloon, ReShape Duo, Elipse, Obalon) are available. However, most information in this section refers to the Orbera.

19.3.1 Indications and Contraindications

The Orbera and other IGB are indicated in association with a specific diet treatment in patients with a history of obesity (at least 5 years) after numerous failures of dietary treatment only or as bridge to surgery [14, 15].

19.3.1.1 Indications
- Grade 1 obese (BMI 30–34.9 kg/m^2) patients with obesity-related comorbidities whose improvement requires mandatory weight loss
- High-risk grade 2–3 obese (BMI 35–49.9 kg/m^2) or superobese (BMI >50 kg/m^2) patients before any other type of surgery (bariatric, orthopedic, cardiac, etc.), as they could benefit from presurgical weight loss to reduce operative risk and incidence of postoperative complications [16].
- Patients who refuse bariatric surgical procedures to help them achieve satisfactory weight loss or, at least, weight stability
- Presurgical tests to evaluate compliance with a pre-established diet program by candidates for restrictive surgery and whose eating behavior is difficult to pinpoint. At the moment, there are no specific limitations as regards age, so the device can be used in children.

19.3.1.2 Contraindications
- Voluminous hiatal hernia (>5 cm);
- Esophagitis (>grade II)
- Duodenal ulcer
- Potential bleeding conditions of the upper gastrointestinal tract
- Outcomes of prior major surgical operations on the gastrointestinal tract and/or certified adhesion syndrome
- Neoplasias
- Chronic treatment with gastric irritants or anticoagulants
- Major or noncollaborative psychiatric disorders
- Alcohol or drug dependence
- Certified pregnancy
- All inflammatory pathologies of the gastrointestinal tract (e.g., Crohn's disease)

19.3.2   Preoperative Workup

All patients should undergo the following clinical tests before IGB placement.
- Complete blood test
- Echocardiogram (ECG) and cardiologic video
- Diagnostic esophagogastroduodenoscopy with *Helicobacter pylori* (HP) analysis to rule out contraindications to balloon placement
- Endocrinological and dietary examinations to exclude endocrine-based obesity
- Psychiatric clinical evaluation to exclude major or noncollaborative psychiatric diseases and to ascertain the presence and the type of the eating disorders (e.g., sweet eating, binge eating disorders, etc.)

In superobese patients (BMI >50 kg/m^2) with breathing distress or in high-risk obese patients (regardless of BMI), chest X-ray, respiratory function tests, and anesthesiologic examination are recommended

19.3.3   Placement and Removal Technique

Orbera/BIB placement and removal can be performed with the patient under conscious sedation with diazepam or midazolam (80%), under unconscious sedation with propofol (15%), or by orotracheal intubation (5%). During placement, the patient is in left lateral decubitus and a diagnostic esophagogastroduodenoscopy is performed. Then, the balloon is positioned with the valve under the cardia and filled under endoscopic vision with 500–700 mL of physiological solution and 10ml vital staining solution (methylene blue). The connection catheter is removed and the valve checked for possible leaks. Mean duration of the procedure is 12 min. Methylene blue is used for early identification of balloon rupture or valve leaks. Should either occur, the solution will be absorbed and will color the urine blue. For this reason, before discharge from the hospital, it is important to sensitize the patient to ongoing urine observation. A diligent anamnesis is essential to exclude the presence of glucose-6-phosphate dehydrogenase (G6PDH) deficit. Patients with this disease, like those afflicted with favism, may experience a hemolytic crisis due to the methylene blue. In these cases, the dye cannot be used and possible balloon rupture or valve leaks can be ascertained by echograph. BIB removal is carried out after 6 months. Due to the delayed gastric emptying achieved with the balloon, the removal procedure should be preceded by a 72-h no roughage diet and by a 24-h semiliquid diet (yoghurt, mashed potatoes, puréed vegetables). It is very important that the patient respect this diet in order to avoid *ab ingestis*, chiefly when the procedure is performed under unconscious sedation. In these cases, the patient should never lose the cough reflex.

The procedure foresees esophagogastroduodenoscopy to facilitate identification of the balloon and its subsequent deflation with a specific device. The BIB is removed when completely deflated using a dedicated grasper. Stomach observation is necessary to exclude possible mucosal lesions. BIB placement can be performed on inpatients, outpatients, and in day hospitals; in Italy, to claim refunding from the National Health Service, is it usually carried out on inpatients with at least 2 days of hospitalization. When performed on an outpatient basis or in day hospitals, the patient must always be properly informed as to adverse symptoms that may arise. It is essential, moreover, that close, ongoing follow-up be carried to facilitate diagnosis and treat complications that may arise, such as hydroelectrolytic imbalance or gastric dilation.

19.3.4 Postplacement Pharmacological Treatment

Due to the secondary effects deriving from the presence of the IGB (nausea, regurgitation or vomiting, cramp-like epigastric pains) and due to the almost total impossibility to eat, during the first 24–36 h after balloon placement, all patients must receive supportive treatment comprising infusion of electrolytic solutions, proton pump inhibitors, and antispasmodic and antiemetic drugs.

19.3.5 Postplacement Diet

The first day foresees a liquid diet only. From the second and up to the sixth or seventh day, a semiliquid diet (yoghurt, mashed potatoes, puréed vegetables) is allowed. The dietetic regime to be associated with the intragastric balloon has not yet been fully standardized. However, by the seventh or eighth day, our patients receive a diet program prepared by the nutritionists, which foresees a daily intake of ~1000–1200 Kcal: 68 g protein (at least 1 g/kg ideal weight), 18 g lipids, 146 g glucides consumed over three main meals and two snacks. For the first 3 months, moreover, a multivitamin supplement is added. This dietetic regime is maintained until BIB removal. Our experience shows that daily consumption of a high volume of vegetables is inadvisable because they are difficult to digest, thus clogging the gastric cavity and inducing vomiting. It is therefore advisable to prescribe vegetables in soup form.

19.3.6 Follow-Up

All patients are contacted by phone every day for the first 7 days. On the 8th day, they undergo an in-office clinical–nutritional examination. During the remaining period, every 2 weeks, the undergoes alternately a clinical–nutritional examination and an evaluation carried out by one of the team of physicians who performed the procedure. Psychological assistance for the entire treatment (6 months) is performed only if requested – either by the patient or the psychologist – during the first pretreatment workup meeting. When there are signs (e.g., blue urine) or symptoms indicating a possible complication, an immediate clinical evaluation, and possibly an esophagogastroduodenoscopy, is essential. Decubital ulcers or gastrectasia indicate the need to remove the BIB.

Before discharge, the patient is made aware of the importance of optimum hydration, as well as ongoing urine checks in order to diagnose in time premature BIB rupture or a possible valve leak. All patients are informed of the increased chance of balloon rupture if it remains in the gastric cavity for longer than the prescribed 6 months.

At the end of the 6th month the BIB will be removed. Then, the following alternatives are evaluated: (a) starting the patient of on a maintenance diet program; (b) consensual placement of a second BIB (multiple treatment); (c) performing a previously planned bariatric surgery.

19.3.7 Outcomes

19.3.7.1 Weight Loss and Impact on Comorbidities

To date, the largest experience with Orbera/BIB was published in 2005 [17] by the Italian Lap-Band and BIB group (GILB). In that study of 2,515 patients with a mean initial BMI of 44.4 kg/m^2 and a mean excess weight of 59.5 kg, a mean BMI loss of 4.9 kg/m^2 and mean %EWL of 33.9% were achieved. Consistently, 6-month treatment demonstrated its effectiveness in resolving or improving obesity-related comorbidities in 44.3 and 44.8% of patients, respectively, while no changes were reported in 10.9%. These data are similar to those registered in our own experience of 1596 placements in 1503 patients from 1998 to 2013; at the end of the treatment, patients showed a mean BMI loss of 7.1 kg/m^2 and a mean %EWL of 34.4%. In our series, weight loss was greater than diet alone [18] and drastically affected the progression of obesity-related diseases, with a resolution or improvement of hypertension, visceral fat and liver volume [19], dyslipidemia, sleep apnea, and joint disease in 90, 86, 80 and 61%, respectively. Moreover, Orbera/BIB is a repeatable treatment. In fact, in a study published by our group, patients who received two consecutive intragastric balloon treatments achieved significantly better postintervention weight loss than those who followed a 7-month diet program after balloon removal [20]. These data are supported by Lopez-Nava et al., who showed that patients continue to lose weight following the second balloon treatment. Data concerning long-term weight-loss outcomes [21] are encouraging. Within the framework of our experience from 1998 to 2006, we retrospectively evaluated weight-loss outcomes in 45 patients with a 60-month follow-up after balloon removal. The rate of success, intended as an %EWL>25%, was 69% at the time of intragastric balloon removal and 30% after 60 months. In addition, investigating the association between long-term weight-loss outcome results and other factors such as initial BMI, age, and sex, factors predicting long-term success were female gender, age <35 years, and initial BMI 35–40 kg/m^2.

Data from GILB showed that diabetic patients undergoing IGB treatment achieved disease resolution or improvement in 32.8 and 54.8% of patients, respectively. Consistently, high rates of resolution or improvement of metabolic syndrome, hypertension, hypertriglyceridemia, type 2 diabetes mellitus, and hypercholesterolemia have been registered in different studies after balloon placement. The metabolic impact of intragastric balloon seems to be maintained in patients whose weight loss percentage 1 year after balloon removal is >10% and has been ascribed mainly to the weight-loss-related decrease in insulin resistance. However, these changes seem to occur earlier in obese (BMI <40 kg/m^2) than in morbidly obese patients (BMI >40 kg/m^2) despite a similar weight loss, as shown by Mirošević et al. [22]. The authors speculated difference may be explained by lower adipose tissue mass and consequent lower leptin and proinflammatory cytokine levels.

19.3.8 Complications (According to Clavien-Dindo Classification)

IGB treatment has acceptable complication rates [23]. Data from the Italian experience with BIB/Orbera, accounting for 3252 patients, showed that the overall incidence of complications was 3.1% (103 patients) [24].

19.3.8.1 Major Complications (Grades III–IV)
The Italian study reported that 32 patients (0.9%) experienced major complications:
–   gastric obstruction (19; 0.58%) requiring balloon removal in 16 cases
–   gastric ulceration (5; 0.15%)
–   gastric perforation (5; 0.15%); four patients had previously undergone surgery: three at the gastric level (Nissen fundoplication, vertical gastroplasty, and gastric band removal because of intragastric migration) and one due to prior thoracic-abdominal trauma. Three patients were managed surgically; two patients (0.06%) died.

19.3.8.2 Minor Complications (Grades I–II)
The Italian study also reported the following minor complications in 71 patients:
–   psychological intolerance (13; 0.9%) requiring early balloon removal
–   esophagitis (39; 1.2%) diagnosed during balloon removal and probably due to the discontinuation of proton pump inhibitors (PPI).

Although device breakage occurred in 19 patients (0.58%), it is important to emphasize that 17 of these patients did not undergo balloon removal within the 6-months period, as advised by the manufacturer.

19.3.9   Latest-Generation Devices

A new class of balloons on the market are procedureless balloons that require no endoscopy for placement or, in some instances, removal.

- Elipse IGB (Allurion Technologies, Wellesley, MA, USA) is an encapsulated polyurethane balloon containing a small radiopaque ring and is easily swallowed by the patient. The capsule is attached to a thin catheter ~75-cm long through which it is filled. Balloon position is checked radiologically to confirm accurate placement prior to filling with 550 mL of fluid, following which the catheter removed. After 4 months, the valve dissolves, the liquid is released, and the balloon is evacuated spontaneously. Due to the newness of the product, detailed information regarding safety and efficacy is as yet unavailable.

- The ReShape Duo (Reshape Medical Inc, San Clemente, CA, USA) comprises two independent balloons of 450-mL capacity each and connected by a flexible tube so that inadvertent deflation of one does not affect the other.

- The Spatz adjustable balloon system (Spatz FGIA Inc, Great Neck, NY, USA) has an extractable tube that allows volume adjustment while the balloon is in the stomach.

- The Obalon gastric balloon (Obalon Therapeutics Inc, San Diego, CA, USA) is packed in a gelatin capsule, then connected to a thin catheter. The capsule is swallowed, and once in the stomach, the gelatin dissolves, freeing the balloon that, after fluoroscopic control, is inflated through the catheter, which is then detached and removed. Up to three balloons can be ingested sequentially depending on the desired hunger control and weight loss. It is endoscopically removed after 12–26 weeks.

Other space-occupying devices are also available, such as the silicone TransPyloric Shuttle (BAROnova Inc, Goleta, CA, USA), which delays gastric emptying with intermittent closures of the pylorus, exploiting peristalsis movement. Another is the Full Sense Device (BFKW LLC, Grand Rapids, MI, USA), a gastroesophageal stent that induces satiety by the pressure it applies on the cardia. Data regarding the safety and efficacy of these novel nonsurgical approaches is still required.

References

1. Ogden CL, Carroll MD, Kit BK, Flegal KM (2014) Prevalence of childhood and adult obesity in the United States, 2011–2012. JAMA 311:806–814
2. Cawley J, Meyerhoefer C (2012) The medical care costs of obesity: an instrumental variables approach. J Health Econ 31:219–230
3. Knowler WC, Barrett-Connor E, Fowler SE (2002) Reduction in the incidence of type 2 diabetes with lifestyle intervention or metformin. N Engl J Med 346:393–403
4. Diabetes Prevention Program Research Group, Knowler WC, Fowler SE et al (2009) 10-year follow-up of diabetes incidence and weight loss in the Diabetes Prevention Program Outcomes Study. Lancet 374:1677–1686

5. Wadden TA, Foreyt JP, Foster GD et al (2011) Weight loss with naltrexone SR/bupropion SR combination therapy as an adjunct to behavior modification: the COR-BMOD trial. Obesity 19:110–120

6. Chang SH, Stoll CR, Song J et al (2014) The effectiveness and risks of bariatric surgery: an updated systematic review and meta-analysis, 2003–2012. JAMA 149:275–287

7. ASGE Bariatric Endoscopy Task Force, Sullivan S, Kumar N et al (2015) ASGE position statement on endoscopic bariatric therapies in clinical practice. Gastrointest Endosc 82:767–772

8. ASGE Bariatric Endoscopy Task Force and ASGE Technology Committee, Abu Dayyeh BK, Kumar N et al (2015) ASGE Bariatric Endoscopy Task Force systematic review and meta-analysis assessing the ASGE PIVI thresholds for adopting endoscopic bariatric therapies. Gastrointest Endosc 82:425–438

9. Jensen MD, Ryan DH, Apovian CM et al (2014) 2013 AHA/ACC/TOS guideline for the management of overweight and obesity in adults: a report of the American College of Cardiology/American Heart Association Task Force on Practice Guidelines and The Obesity Society. J Am Coll Cardiol 63:2985–3023

10. ASGE Bariatric Endoscopy Task Force; ASGE Technology Committee, Abu Dayyeh BK et al (2015) Endoscopic bariatric therapies. Gastrointest Endosc 81:1073–1086

11. Lopez-Nava G, Galvao MP, da Bautista-Castano I, Jimenez A et al (2015) Endoscopic sleeve gastroplasty for the treatment of obesity. Endoscopy 47:449–452

12. Sharaiha RZ, Kedia P, Kumta N et al (2015) Initial experience with endoscopic sleeve gastroplasty: technical success and reproducibility in the bariatric population. Endoscopy 47:164–166

13. ASGE/ASMBS Task Force on Endoscopic Bariatric Therapy (2011) A pathway to endoscopic bariatric therapies. Surg Obes Relat Dis 7:672–682

14. Weiner R, Gutberlet H, Bockhorn H (1999) Preparation of extremely obese patients for laparoscopic gastric banding by gastric-balloon therapy. Obes Surg 9:261–264

15. Genco A, Lorenzo M, Baglio G et al (2014) Does the intragastric balloon have a predictive role in subsequent LAP-BAND surgery? Italian multicenter study results at 5-year follow-up. Surg Obes Relat Dis 10:474–478

16. Pasulka PS, Bistrian BR, Benotti PN et al (1986) The risks of surgery in obese patients. Ann Intern Med 104:540–546

17. Genco A, Bruni T, Doldi SB et al (2005) Bioenterics intragastric balloon: the Italian experience with 2,515 patients. Obes Surg 15:1161–1164

18. Genco A, Balducci S, Bacci V et al (2008) Intragastric balloon or diet alone? A retrospective evaluation. Obes Surg 18:989–992

19. Busetto L, Tregnaghi A, De Marchi F et al (2002) Liver volume and visceral obesity in women with hepatic steatosis undergoing gastric banding. Obes Res 10:408–411

20. Genco A, Cipriano M, Bacci V et al (2010) Intragastric balloon followed by diet vs intragastric balloon followed by another balloon: a prospective study on 100 patients. Obes Surg 20:1496–1500

21. Genco A, Maselli R, Cipriano M et al (2013) Long-term multiple intragastric balloon treatment: a new strategy to treat morbid obese patients refusing surgery. Prospective 6-year follow-up study. Obes Surg 23:1067–1068

22. Mirošević G, Nikolić M, Kruljac I et al (2014) Decrease in insulin resistance has a key role in improvement of metabolic profile during intragastric balloon treatment. Endocrine 45:331–334

23. Dumonceau JM (2008) Evidence-based review of the Bioenterics intragastric balloon for weight loss. Obes Surg 18:1611–1617

24. Genco A; Furbetta F; Micheletto G et al (2007) The Italian experience of 3,252 patients treated by Bioenterics Intragastric Balloon (BIB) In: Italian Society for the Surgery of Obesity. Abstracts of the 14th National Congress (Florence, Italy, October 1–3, 2006). Obes Surg 17:130

Other Bariatric Procedures

20

Marcello Lucchese, Stefano Cariani, Enrico Amenta,
Ludovico Docimo, Salvatore Tolone, Francesco Furbetta,
Giovanni Lesti, and Marco Antonio Zappa

20.1   Introduction

Bariatric surgery can still be considered a "young" surgery in its continuous evolution, even though the first surgical procedure was performed 70 years ago [1]. Surgical pioneers developed innovative procedures that initially caused malabsorption only, then restricted volume intake, and eventually both techniques were combined [2]. Variations, alterations, and modifications of these original procedures, combined with the concept of weight-loss surgery that eventually became known as metabolic surgery, are the demonstration of this continuous surgical improvement.

The intense efforts to follow and document outcomes after bariatric procedures have led to the evolution of modern bariatric surgery. Many authors have developed different technical solutions to solve some of the problems with what is considered standard procedures.

One such procedure is the Roux-en-Y gastric bypass on vertical banded gastroplasty (RYGB on VBG), a variation of the standard RYGB, with the goal of developing a gastric bypass allowing exploration of the excluded stomach and biliary tract [3, 4]. A similar procedure associated with resection of the gastric fundus was also proposed [5].

Intragastric balloon (IGB) and adjustable gastric banding (AGB) have been proposed as sequential systematic treatments to achieve a degree of weight loss before a definitive RYGB procedure [6].

Even in the malabsorptive procedures, some alternative procedures have been proposed. Hallberg proposed a modification of the jejunoileal bypass by adding anastomosis of the excluded intestinal tract with the gallbladder, thus

M. Lucchese (✉)
General, Metabolic and Emergency Unit, Department of Surgery, Santa Maria Nuova Hospital
Florence, Italy
e-mail: mlucch@iol.it

L. Angrisani (Ed), Bariatric and Metabolic Surgery,
Updates in Surgery
DOI: 10.1007/ 978-88-470-3944-5_20, © Springer-Verlag Italia 2017

avoiding postoperative diarrhea due to dramatic reduction in the absorption of biliary juice [7–10].

In this chapter, we present some bariatric procedures that are still considered alternative because, although they have been published in the literature, they are not performed universally, but are regularly performed in some centers, and follow-up results are reported for many patients. In the following paragraphs these procedures are presented by the authors who first proposed the technique or by surgeons regularly performing it.

20.2   Biliointestinal Bypass

The biliointestinal bypass (BIBP) is a malabsorptive procedure. Indications and limits of this technique are those commonly adopted for this category of bariatric procedures. The BIBP was introduced into clinical practice by Hallberg [7] and Eriksson [11] in the late 1970s, as a modification of the jejunoileal bypass. The aim was to reduce the side effects linked with the bypassed limb. The technical peculiarity of BIBP involves an anastomosis between the gallbladder and the proximal stump of the excluded jejunal limb (Fig. 20.1)

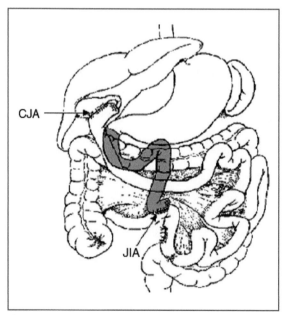

Fig. 20.1 Biliointestinal bypass (BIBP) with cholecystojejunal anastomosis (CJA) and jejunoileal anastomosis (JIA) (reproduced with permission from [12])

20.2.1 Surgical Technique

The BIBP can be performed with the laparoscopic (usually four to six trocars, according to surgeon's preference) or open approach. The BIBP consists of the following steps (Fig. 20.1): Identification of the duodenojejunal flexure (D-J flexure, or Treitz ligament); measurement of the small bowel from a point marking the first 30 cm of jejunum; measurement of the last 12–18 cm of ileum starting from the ileocecal valve; section of the jejunum 30 cm from the D-J flexure; side-to side jejunoileal anastomosis 12–18 cm from the ileocecal valve; cholecystojejunal anastomosis (with possible removal of gallstones through the surgical access to the gallbladder for anastomosis), using a linear mechanical stapler (30 or 45). In our experience, we opt for a less malabsorptive BIBP, sectioning the jejunum 40 cm distal to the Treitz ligament and anastomosing it to 40 cm proximal to the ileocecal valve. BIBP strength lies in its total reversibility in case of failure or complications due to malabsorption. Moreover, this is the only malabsorptive procedure in which the stomach is not resected; therefore, a restrictive intervention can be considered as a revisional procedure in case of failed weight loss. At the same time, the duodenum and main bile duct can be explored with standard endoscopic procedures, if required, since the intestinal bypass involves the small bowel distal to the papilla.

20.2.2 Rationale for the Procedure

BIBP creates nutrient malabsorption by reducing the absorbing surface (considering an alimentary limb of 45–80 cm, plus the duodenum) and thus accelerates transit. The cholecystojejunal anastomosis diverts a large portion of the bile, thus reducing the absorption of lipids. Theoretically, bile washout in the excluded limb can also prevent the formation of gallstones and bacterial overgrowth while assuring enterohepatic bile-salt circulation. All these features lead to a lower number of bowel movements per day and the dramatic decrease of serious complications related to jejunoileal bypass. Furthermore, BIBP does not expose the patient to the risk of anemia related to a deficiency of intrinsic factors (since the stomach and last portion of the ileum are entirely preserved), and a small residual flow of bile though the duodenum can guarantee satisfactory absorption of vitamins A, D, E, and K.

20.2.3 Results

In a multicenter Italian series [13] consisting of 1030 patients, the average weight loss after 1 year was reported to be 14–33% of initial weight, with body mass index (BMI) loss of 18–35%. These results were confirmed by authors' experience [10] with 347 obese patients. Weight loss reach a plateau within 18–24 months after surgery, with a percentage of excess weight loss (%EWL) of 60–70%. Weight loss remained >60% at 5-year follow-up; 2.5–5% of patients experience insufficient weight loss. In the first months after surgery, diarrhea occurred approximately five to seven times a day. After weight stabilization, bowel movements occurred two to three times day on average.

BIBP causes a drastic reduction in serum levels of cholesterol and triglycerides, which remains constant over the years. In the first postoperative months, there is a significant increase in liver enzymes glutamic oxaloacetic transminase (GOT) and glutamate pyruvic transaminase (GPT), indicating liver overload. These values begin to normalize in the third month after surgery due to better liver function, which entails a reduction of hepatic overload itself. All diseases related to obesity and the metabolic syndrome show a dramatic improvement or a complete remission [8]. In particular, glycemic control improves markedly and therefore drastically reduces the need for drugs or insulin. Remission was recently reported in 83% of cases with type 2 diabetes mellitus (T2DM) preoperatively [10].

20.2.4 Complications

20.2.4.1 Early Complications
BIBP is burdened with complications within the first postoperative month by the same rate of complications described for all abdominal surgery involving intestinal anastomoses (i.e., bleeding, leaks, infections). The reported mortality rate is ~0.5–1%. The most frequent complication is represented by inflammation (~68% of cases). Severe diarrhea, due to dietary restrictions in most cases, appears more rarely and is accompanied by electrolyte imbalances and requires appropriate infusional nutritional support. If not treated, diarrhea can also cause perianal abscesses and fistulas [9].

20.2.4.2 Late Complications
Cholelithiasis appears in ~4% of patients. It can be treated medically using dissolving therapy with bile acid analogs), although in most cases, it is due to cholecystojejunal anastomotic stenosis, which requires surgical revision using a laparoscopic approach. Oxalic nephrolithiasis (5.3%) is caused by an inappropriate diet. Abdominal colicky pain due to altered gut microbiota and consequent gas formation and migrant polyarthralgias affecting distal joints is episodic (4.3%). The recurrent abdominal pain is treated successfully in most cases with a course of antibiotics orally. Protein malnutrition is rare but is usually due to inadequate protein intake or absorption and electrolyte malabsorption. These complications are serious and require intensive medical treatment and sometimes intravenous nutritional support and revisional surgery [10].

20.3   Roux-en-Y Gastric Bypass on Vertical Banded Gastroplasty

Roux-en-Y gastric bypass on vertical banded gastroplasty (RYGB-on-VBG), is a technique derived from the standard RYGB with the goal of creating a gastric bypass in which it is possible to perform a standard endoscopic and an oral contrast study of the excluded stomach. The concept was conceived in 2002 after a pilot study performed with a functional gastric bypass with the same aim [14, 15]. In the midterm, the RYGB-on-VBG procedure reached similar outcomes as the standard techniques of gastric bypass both in terms of weight loss and incidence of surgical complications [3]. Moreover, it demonstrated similar good results when performed in other bariatric centers, thus proving to be highly standardized and reproducible while enabling diagnostic evaluation of the bypassed stomach and biliary tract [4]. Progressively, outcomes of RYGB-on-VBG have been publicly presented and discussed in international meetings [16–18]. Similar results were obtained when used as a revisional procedure after failure of previous restrictive techniques [19]. Long-term results following RYGB-on-VBG are available as from a single-center experience [16], that at present has a 12-year clinical follow-up.

While achieving weight loss outcomes as good as to those after the standard procedure, RYGB-on-VBG enables traditional diagnostic evaluation of the bypassed stomach [20]. Although RYGB-on-VBG is technically more demanding than standard RYGB, the low rate of early and late complications suggests considering the procedure in selected patients with chronic conditions in the gastric remnant, in whom it is advisable to avoid creating blind, unexplorable sections of the digestive tract.

20.3.1 Surgical Technique

The definitive technique of RYGB-on-VBG has already been described [3]. In brief, gastric pouch construction is fashioned as during the Mason/MacLean VBG, with a gastrojejunostomy (2 cm in diameter) to a 150-cm Roux-en-Y limb performed proximally to the pouch outlet (1 cm in diameter). The outlet is encircled with a soft polytetrafluoroethylene (PTFE) band to prevent enlargement of the passage between the pouch and the remnant (Fig. 20.2). The gastric outlet inner diameter is standardized over a 38-Ch endogastric tube. Initially, the RYGB-on-VBG was performed using only the open approach; in 2009, using the laparoscopic approach also became an option [21].

20.3.2 Outcomes

According to the most recent data of a single-center experience [15] – presently based on 456 patients who received a RYGB-on-VBG as primary operation from

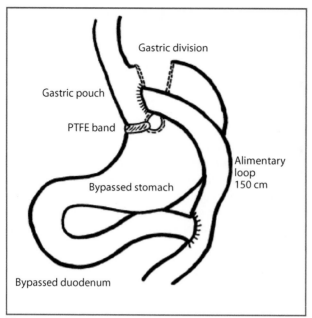

Fig. 20.2: Roux-en-Y gastric bypass on vertical banded gastroplasty: latest technique

2002 to 2015 – mean preoperative BMI was48 ± 8.5 kg/m² (%EBW 99 ± 36.2%). Mean overall dropout rate was 10%. Thus, the number of patients eligible for data analysis was 450 after 6 months and 380, 290, 213, 187, 149, and 63 after 1, 2, 5, 7, 9, and 12 years, respectively. At 1 year after surgery, mean %EWL was 67% and decreased slightly to 60% at 12 years. An upper gastrointestinal endoscopy, when required, was possible in all patients who had prior RYGB-on-VBG (Table 20.1).

Table 20.1 Roux-en-Y gastric bypass on vertical banded gastroplasty (RYGB-on-VBG). Results 2002-2015

	Surgery	6 months	1 year	2 years	5 years	7 years	9 years	12 years
Number of patients	456	450	380	290	213	187	149	63
Mean BMI (SD)	48.0 (8.5)	34.8 (6.5)	30.8 (6.0)	31.0 (5.3)	31.4 (6.0)	32.3 (6.1)	32.5 (6.1)	33.0 (6.0)
Mean %EWL (SD)	–	55.4 (16.8)	67.4 (18.1)	69.2 (17.9)	67.8 (18.4)	65.1 (17.8)	62.3 (16.6)	60.1 (20.5)

RYGB-on-VBG Roux-en-Y gastric bypass on vertical banded gastroplasty, *BMI* body mass index (kg/m²), *%EWL* percentage excess weight loss, *SD* standard deviation

20.3.3 Complications

Six patients (1.3%) had surgical treatment for early complications (Clavien-Dindo grade IIIb); mortality was 0.6% following two grade IVa and one grade IVb medical complication. Late complications were seven (1.5%) band erosions (four patients had surgical revision), five (1%) vertical staple-line disruption (three patients had surgical revision), and four (0.8%) anastomotic ulcers [treated with proton pump inhibitors (PPI)].

20.4   Roux-en-Y Gastric Bypass with Fundectomy and Explorable Stomach

Most bariatric surgeons consider the standard laparoscopic Roux-en-Y gastric bypass (LRYGB) the ideal procedure for treating severe obesity. The problem with this procedure is that the bypassed stomach cannot be explored, and thus there is no opportunity to diagnose and treat diseases of the stomach, duodenum, and main bile duct. In March 2001, Lesti developed a model of gastric bypass, making subsequent modifications up to the final version used since January 2007. The current model of LRYGB with fundectomy and explorable stomach [LRYGB(FES)], in which the gastric fundus is removed, is based on the use of a device that allows the stomach to be isolated from passage of the food bolus but also to remain examinable by endoscopy, providing diagnostic and/or operative possibilities. (Fig. 20.3). The reversible LRYGB(FES) has similar results to the standard model. Removing the gastric fundus leads to a marked decrease

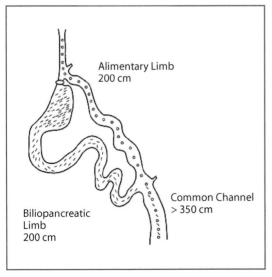

Fig. 20.3 Roux-en-Y gastric bypass with fundectomy (Lesti's technique)

Alimentary Limb
200 cm

Common Channel
> 350 cm

Biliopancreatic
Limb
200 cm

of ghrelin, a hormone that increases the sense of hunger, and to an increase in peptide tyrosine-tyrosine (PYY) and glucagonlike peptide-1 (GLP-1), hormones that block hunger and play an important role in controlling diabetes.

20.4.1 Surgical Technique

This laparoscopic procedure is done with four 10- to 12-mm trocars and one 5-mm trocar. The gastrocolic ligament, opened at Van Goethem's point, is sectioned toward the angle of His: attention is paid to cutting the short vessels. A 36-Fr bougie is introduced into the stomach, and the linear stapler–cutter device is fired beginning at Van Goethem's point at the great curvature toward the lesser curvature 7 cm from the cardias. Three firings of the stapler parallel to the bougie are applied to make the pouch as narrow as possible (20–30 mL). An expanded polytetrafluoroethylene (ePTFE) band 1-mm thick, 5- to 7-cm long, and 1-cm wide is placed 7 cm from the cardias to gently close the end of the pouch. The mean length of the ePTFE band is 57 mm (range 53–65 mm). The jejunum, identified at the Treitz ligament and followed distally for 200–220 cm, is pulled cephalad toward the gastric pouch in the antecolic position after separation of the greater omentum.

The gastrojejunal anastomosis is made side to side, 2.5- to 3-cm wide in the posterior wall of the pouch, starting 5 cm from the cardias, using an endocutter blue cartridge (Echelon). The jejunumileum anastomosis is made 200–220 cm from the pouch, side to side, 2.5- to 3-cm wide. Lesti's technique includes a long biliary limb: first, because the gastroanastomosis is made substantially with the last part of the jejunum, that is very important for the theory of hindgut incretin secretion; second, because in the case of failure, it is very easy to convert the procedure into a long distal gastric bypass. The common channel was >350 cm in all cases.

Mean operative time was 152 (108–227) min, postoperative stay was 4.74 (3–8) days, and operative mortality zero The only early postoperative complication was one important intra-abdominal bleeding occurring on the second postoperative day, which required open surgery; the point of bleeding was not found. Two cases of internal hernia occurred after 3 and 25 months, respectively; both revisions were performed laparoscopically without complications. No leak, migration, ulcer, or stricture occurred in either the early or late follow-up, and there were no minor complications during the 60 months of follow-up.

20.4.2 Outcomes

We report the results of 454 severely obese patients who underwent a LRYGB(FES) with the ePTFE band between January 2007 and December 2014 [5]. All patients were selected according to criteria for bariatric surgery proposed by the US National Institutes of Health (NIH) Consensus of 1991 and replicated and updated by the Italian Society of Obesity Surgery (SICOB) Patients eligible for bariatric surgery (BMI >40 kg/m² or BMI >35 kg/m² with obesity-related comorbidities) underwent evaluation by a multidisciplinary bariatric team at our center for obesity disorders. The population comprised 288 women and 166 men with a mean age of 43.6 (range 27–68) years and a preoperative BMI of 48.2 (range 36.7–58.3) kg/m², weight 136,48 (range 98.3–158.5) kg, and excess weight 58.2 (range 34.5–7.2) kg. Existing comorbidities were T2DM 24.2%, arterial hypertension 31.3%, metabolic syndrome 21.9%, obstructive sleep apnea syndrome 26,4%, depression 15.8%, and gastroesophageal reflux 36.4%. At 5-years follow-up, resolution was seen in T2DM 68.5%, hypertension 67.4%, obstructive sleep apnea syndrome 60.5%, gastroesophageal reflux 84.8%; improvement was seen in T2DM 21.4%, hypertension 26.1%, obstructive sleep apnea syndrome 39.5%, gastroesophageal reflux 15.2%, and arthritis 100%. The % EWL at 1 year in 414 was 77.8%, at 3 years in 278 patients 84.4%, and at 5 years in 166 patients 79.6%. Preoperatively, BMI was 48.2 kg/m² and at 5 years 30.7 kg/m², with a mean loss of 17.5 kg/m².

20.5   Functional Gastric Bypass

The functional gastric bypass (FGB) is consistent with laparoscopic adjustable gastric banding (LAGB), which creates the pouch of a long-limb gastric bypass when fully inflated. The aim of the procedure is to obtain complete diversion of food into the alimentary limb, with the band fully inflated, while allowing band deflation to balance efficacy and to allow access to the excluded stomach with a standard endoscope if necessary (diagnostic-operative in case of suspicion of any pathology arising from the gastric remnant or biliary tree). The design of this technique excludes blind tracts due to band adjustability. The presented technique was devised and has been developed by Francesco Furbetta since its first application and description in 2001 [22].

20.5.1   Surgical Technique

The LAGB is placed across the cardia following the pars flaccida or perigastric technique (Fig. 20.4). An antecolic gastrojejunal anastomosis on the gastric pouch is fashioned through a double-layer hand-sewn technique. Roux-en-Y limb lengths are measured under tension from the ileocecal valve to create a 200-cm alimentary limb and a 150-cm common limb, depending on the pouch size [22].

20.5.2   How it Works: Safety and Efficacy

Food restriction is achieved with an adjustable small pouch; a large gastrojejunal anastomosis (≥15 mm) maximizes the metabolic effect of the distal gastric bypass

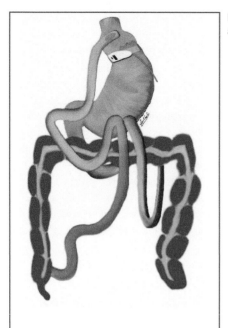

Fig. 20.4 Functional gastric bypass (FGB) according to Furbetta

with the lowest possible risk of malabsorption. It is also possible to switch food passage from the gastric bypass to the gastric remnant, just by deflating the band. As a revisional procedure, the functional bypass could improve the restrictive mechanism of the gastric band, adding metabolic efficacy through a long limb adjustable bypass. Thus, patients can undergo a procedure that can be adapted to their individual characteristics [22].

20.5.3 Results and complications

From January 2001 to October 2015, in this monocentric experience, the FGB was performed on 209 patients: in 155 out of 3050 patients with a previous LAGB and in 54 cases, as the first surgical step. Long-term efficacy of the procedure was assessed on the 68 eligible patients with a 5-year follow-up. In particular, mean 5-year BMI was 30.7 kg/m^2, corresponding to a %EWL of 52.4% and a BMI loss of 67.5%. Results were achieved with no mortality. Out of the entire group of 209 patients, early complications were consistent with only one anastomotic leak (Clavien-Dindo grade IVa); late complications, represented by erosion, were experienced in 6%.

Even though the procedure lacks widespread application and the main concerns are related to the possible band complications, the FGB procedure brings together the minimally invasive LAGB, the stabilized, different working of the GBP, and the efficacy of the BPD. Their relative characteristics maximize safety and efficacy through reversibility, adjustability, absence of blind limbs, and the sequential treatment opposite to re-do. All this allows scientific and technical progress.

20.6   Conclusions

Despite good results in terms of outcomes and safety of these alternative bariatric procedures, information in the literature remains scarce. However, every alternative or new procedure in bariatric surgery should be considered as being potential valuable. Publication of short- and long-term results of alternative bariatric procedures are required in order to report their safety and efficacy. It is important for surgical societies to recall that procedures such as the sleeve gastrectomy and the so-called mini gastric bypass – which are now practiced worldwide – were initially considered investigational procedures. We believe that continued recognition of different mechanisms of action and new techniques in bariatric surgery will lead to more precise indications and individualization of the best procedure for the best results in each patient.

References

1. Saber AA, Elgamal MH, McLeod MK (2008) Bariatric surgery: the past, present, and future. Obes Surg 18:121–128
2. Lo Menzo E, Szomstein S, Rosenthal RJ (2015) Changing trends in bariatric surgery. Scand J Surg 104:18–23
3. Cariani S, Amenta E (2007) Three-year results of Roux-en-Y gastric bypass-on-vertical banded gastroplasty: an effective and safe procedure which enables endoscopy and X-ray study of the stomach and biliary tract. Obes Surg 17:1312–1318
4. Cariani S, Palandri P, Della Valle E et al (2008) Italian multicenter experience of Roux-en-Y gastric bypass on vertical banded gastroplasty: four-year results of effective and safe innovative procedure enabling traditional endoscopic and radiographic study of bypassed stomach and biliary tract. Surg Obes Relat Dis 4:16–25
5. Lesti G (2015) Tecnica del by-pass gastrico sec. Lesti. Oral communication at XXIII SICOB National Congress, Baveno (Italy)
6. Greve JW, Furbetta F, Lesti G et al (2004) Combination of laparoscopic adjustable gastric banding and gastric bypass: current situation and future prospects: routine use not advised. Obes Surg 14:683–689
7. Hallberg D (1980) A survey of surgical techniques for treatment of obesity and a remark on the bilio-intestinal bypass method. Am J Clin Nutr 33(2 Suppl):499–501
8. Micheletto G, Mozzi E, Lattuada E et al (2007) The bilio-intestinal bypass. Ann Ital Chir 78:27–30
9. Ruggiero R, Docimo G, Russo V et al (2010) Bilio-intestinal bypass in the treatment of metabolic syndrome in obese patient. G Chir 31(11–12):527–533 [Article in Italian]

10. Del Genio G, Gagner M, Limongelli P et al (2015) Remission of type 2 diabetes in patients undergoing biliointestinal bypass for morbid obesity: a new surgical treatment. Surg Obes Relat Dis [Epub ahead of print] doi:10.1016/j.soard.2015.12.003
11. Eriksson F (1981) Biliointestinal bypass. Int J Obes 5:437–447
12. Corradini SG, Eramo A, Lubrano C et al (2005) Comparison of changes in lipid profile after biliointestinal bypass and gastric banding in patients with morbid obesity. Obes Surg 15:367–377
13. Micheletto G, Badiali M, Danelli PG et al (2008) The biliointestinal bypass: a thirty-years experience. Ann Ital Chir 79:419–426 [Article in Italian]
14. Cariani S, Vittimberga G, Grani S et al (2002) Prospective study on functional Roux-en-Y gastric bypass to avoid gastric exclusion. In: IFSO Congress Programme and Abstracts. Obes Surg 12:469
15. Cariani S, Lucchi A, Guerra M, Faccani E, Amenta E (2004) Evolution of functional Roux-en-Y gastric bypass: from adjustable band to Gore-tex band. In: IFSO European Symposium. Obes Surg 14:471
16. Leuratti L, Picariello E, Balsamo F, Cariani S (2012) Long term results after Roux-en-Y gastric bypass on vertical banded gastroplasty with explorable remnant: does the presence of a gastro-gastric outlet impact on final outcomes in term of metabolic efficacy and weight loss? Obes Surg 22:1160
17. Cariani S, Giorgini E, Agostinelli L et al (2009) Mid-term outcomes of Roux-en-Y gastric bypass on vertical banded gastroplasty. Surg Obes Relat Dis 5(3 suppl):S30
18. Cariani S, Leuratti L, Picariello E, Spasari E (2011) An outlet for endoscopic access to the remnant does not reduce the effectiveness of gastric bypass: long-term outcomes of a modified Roux-en-Y gastric bypass that allows traditional endoscopy of bypassed stomach. In: IFSO Congress – Plenary Sessions. Obes Surg 21:1000
19. Cariani S, Agostinelli L, Leuratti L et al (2010) Bariatric revisionary surgery for failed or complicated vertical banded gastroplasty (VBG): Comparison of VBG reoperation (re-VBG) versus Roux-en-Y gastric bypass-on-VBG (RYGB-on-VBG). J Obes 2010 doi:10.1155/2010/206249
20. Leuratti L, Di Simone MP, Cariani S (2013) Unexpected changes in the gastric remnant in asymptomatic patients after Roux-en-Y gastric bypass on vertical banded gastroplasty. Obes Surg 23:131–139
21. Cariani S, Agostinelli L, Giorgini E et al (2009) Open and laparoscopic approach of a new surgical technique, which enables traditional diagnostic evaluation of the bypassed stomach: the Roux-en-Y gastric bypass on vertical banded gastroplasty. In: International Federation for the Surgery of Obesity and metabolic disorders. XIV World Congress. Obes Surg 19:1048
22. Furbetta F, Gambinotti G (2002) Functional gastric bypass with an adjustable gastric band. Obes Surg 12:876–880

Printed in the United States
By Bookmasters